HOW TO

WILD

SWIM

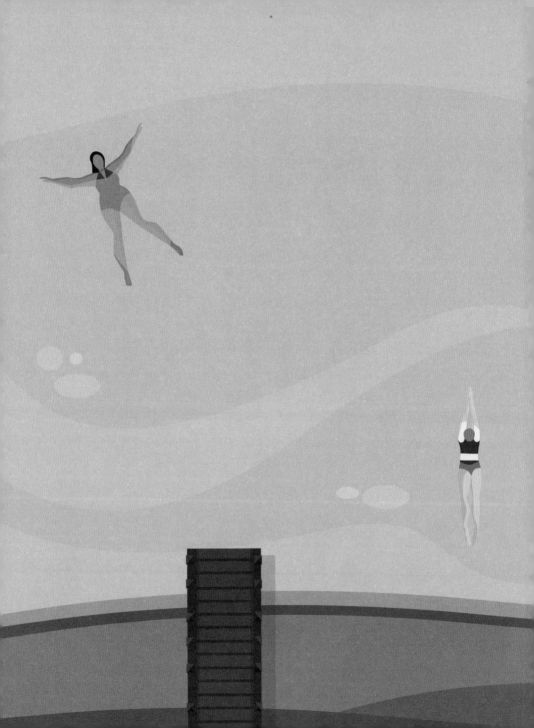

HOW TO

WHAT TO KNOW

WILD

BEFORE TAKING THE PLUNGE

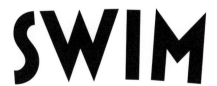

ELLA FOOTE

CONTENTS

Diving in   6

1   Why swim wild?   10
2   Can you swim?   22
3   What to wear   36
4   Swim gear   48
5   Where to swim   66
6   Bodies of water   76
7   Risks! Is it safe?   90
8   Hot and cold conditions   100
9   The seasons and weather   114
10   Preparing to swim   124
11   Swimming strokes and skills   132
12   After-swim care   146

Top 20 places to wild swim   154
Index   156
Further reading   158
Acknowledgments   159

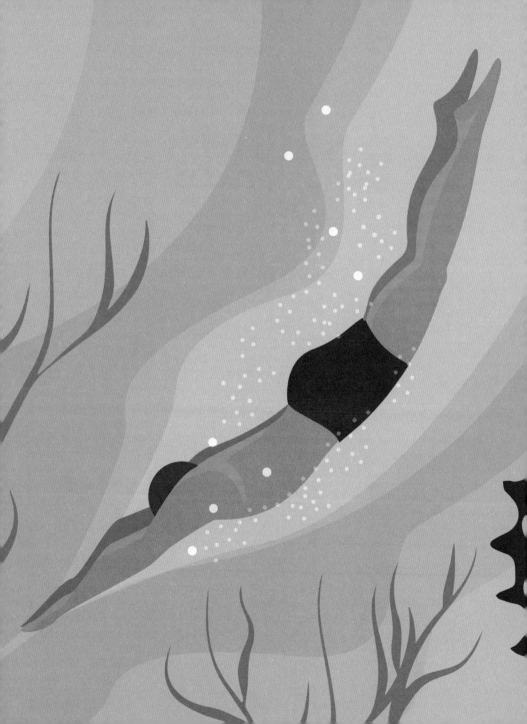

Diving in

Nothing sparks awe and evokes magic quite like swimming wild. It's a sensory experience that encourages childlike play and adventure. Unlike dodging a discarded bandage or untangling someone else's hair from your fingers in an indoor pool, outdoor water tickles you with weeds and reeds. In wild water you encounter wildlife at earth level: duck poo between your toes, and—depending on the time of year—the sweet scent of water mint, damp woody aromas, or musky syrupy smells from flora and fauna. Wild swimming can be restorative, energize you, or offer transformation. Scuffed up shins, salty hair, or muddy feet—nothing makes you feel more feral. Swimming wild is different than just swimming. Outdoor swimming takes some consideration. Where you swim will have a huge impact on how you swim, what you wear, and what to take with you. Unlike life-guarded and often warm swimming pools, open water is natural, ever-changing, and possibly cold. How you find the water today will be different tomorrow, and no swim is ever the same.

While I have always loved the water, I haven't always loved its wild unpredictability or the looming creatures that inhabit it. I came to realize, however, that almost everything in the water is more afraid of you than you are of it—pretty much everything swims or moves away from you. Except for jellyfish—they blob around with currents, tides, and swell and still really bother me! I also didn't understand why people liked river swimming—there are a lot more weeds in rivers than in the sea. But like many things in life, the more you do something, the better you get and the more you learn. The sea will always be a deep first love and joy, my first wild water experience, but I fell in love with river swimming. This has been a slow burn that has become meaningful and essential. I discovered the joy of rushing, bubbling young rivers with deep pools. I found comfort in the reeds brushing my legs and the squidge of mud between my toes. I take great joy in journey swims from one place to another down a river, enjoying the vast widths and lengths ahead of me, and allowing the natural flow to push, float, or pull me downstream. Many sorrows and difficulties have been washed away in a river.

Living away from the sea I had to find water to love inland. As well as rivers, I have sought out lakes, ponds, and outdoor pools. My love of maps extended to being spread out on top of them seeking, searching, and crawling over the paper with my fingers looking for blue wiggles or blue blobs near home or wherever I traveled. After years of training and swimming at events —across channels, down rivers, or looping in

I want to ignite the wild magic and play within all of us to swim feral and free in blue spaces.

lakes—I decided to return to the water for myself. I wanted to rediscover the magic and find new swimming experiences and locations, without the pressure to swim for a set period or distance. I wanted to swim just for joy, head down or head up. I wanted to rewild myself in the water. Around the same time, I changed my work and found a way to share my love of the water through writing, photography, guiding, coaching, and more recently, teaching. All my work today involves wearing a swimsuit. In a week I tackle teaching children in a warm pool, guide clients down rivers or across lakes, and get to put all my experience and connections together into a monthly magazine for outdoor swimmers.

After decades of swimming outdoors and writing columns of words about it in magazines and newspapers, it makes sense to pull this into something more useful. This guide will help rewild you in the water. It aims to answer any questions you may have about whether it is safe, or even allowed, and to reassure you that a simple swimsuit and towel may be all that you need, but also suggests what else to pack for a bigger adventure. I hope to point you in the direction of water you know and desire to dip into, armed with some knowledge to mitigate the risks. But above all, I want to ignite the wild magic and play within all of us to swim feral and free in blue spaces.

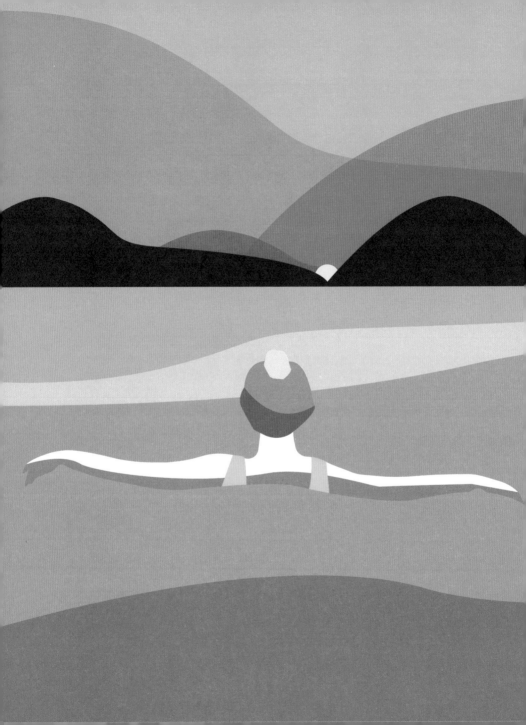

1
WHY SWIM WILD?

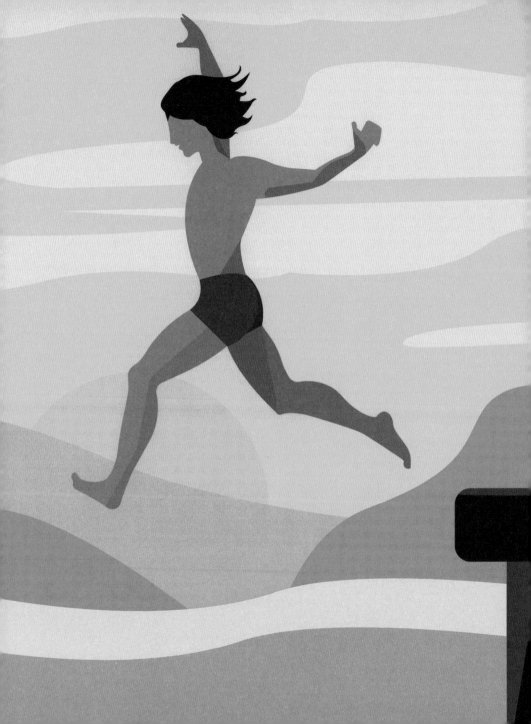

TAKING
THE PLUNGE

Why not take the plunge and try wild swimming? Yes, you might think it will be cold, or a little risky, or not as clean as a swimming pool, but the benefits far outnumber the reasons why you wouldn't want to dip a toe into wilder water.

If you explore the global history of swimming, you'll see it all started outdoors. Karen Eva Carr explains in her book, *Shifting Currents*, that historic evidence shows humans getting into the ocean 165,000 years ago at the southern tip of Africa. In Italy, 100,000 years ago, Neanderthals were diving in

the Mediterranean to retrieve clamshells, their ear bones suggesting that they swam enough to get swimmer's ear, an infection caused by water in the ears. Swimming for pleasure instead of need can be traced back to Old Kingdom Egypt. It was the Egyptians who first inspired the Greeks and Romans to swim, and then the desire to emulate the Greeks and Romans swimming for exercise and medical benefit spread across Europe. Today swimmers across the world plunge into water for spiritual practice, for rehabilitation, and for their physical and mental health.

10 reasons to try wild swimming

1 It is an excellent physical activity

Swimming provides a full-body workout and challenges your cardiovascular system. It has lower injury risk than land-based sport and is effectively used in rehabilitation therapy to aid physical ability and treatment. It is low-impact and gentle, so once you have learnt how to swim, you can swim your whole life. If you take your swimming outside, you increase the benefits. As well as moving your body, you are exposed to natural daylight, breathing fresh air, and engaging with wildlife—all scientifically proven to improve overall health. Cold water increases heart rate, reduces inflammation, and focuses us on our breathing. Swimming releases all the feel-good hormones and endorphins.

2 It improves mental health

As well as a flood of anecdotal evidence in popular culture and the media, many people have shared stories of how outdoor swimming has improved their mental health, cured their depression, or boosted productivity. It has been scientifically proven that we benefit from being outside and beside, or in, water. In her book, *Losing Eden*, Lucy Jones explores the vital link between being outside and the nervous system, immune function, and mood. She explains how negative ions, molecules that are abundant in certain outdoor environments, have been found to activate the release of serotonin, improving mood. Negative ions are more intense around water and in natural areas, which might explain why time spent near rivers, beside the sea, or around waterfalls in the mountains can make us feel so good and lift our spirits. Where air molecules are broken apart by moving water there is an increase in negative ions—the number falls significantly when indoors.

3 It releases your inner child

Wild water is more fun than indoor swimming. It ignites that playful, childlike glee. It feels rebellious and free. It can be meditative and soothing, or social and joyful. When walking beside a river, it is common to find rope tied to tree branches, thrown up by kids wanting to swing and leap into the water below. Sticks are thrown from bridges; we feel compelled to paddle in the shallows or seek surrounding wildlife. Beaches offer sand to build with, rock pools to dip into, shells to collect, and rocks to swim around or leap off. People of all ages are eager to pick up a bit of sea glass or pop a smooth rock into a pocket. Wild water spikes our curiosity like when we were toddlers—ducking and diving down into the water to brush seaweed or peek into corners seeking sea life. Our imagination is ignited; we recount tales of pirates and mermaids. We can feel afraid in deep, dark lakes or in fast-rushing rivers. We are more open to risk and adventure when we swim wild.

Wild water is more fun than indoor swimming. It ignites that playful, childlike glee. It feels rebellious and free.

4 It makes you care more about the environment

Nothing can ground you in the reality of human impact on our environment more than a wild swim. You can see and experience first-hand what litter and pollution can do to wildlife and ecosystems. No one wants to swim in an ocean full of plastic or a river containing sewage. A lakeside picnic and swim can be ruined by a discarded disposable grill or empty beer bottles. Witnessing how fish, birds, and other fauna are forced to adapt or change because of human influence can be the start of action. Outdoor swimmers become protectors of place, guardians of the water, or environmental warriors. In a recent study by *Outdoor Swimmer* magazine, 79 percent of swimmers surveyed have become increasingly concerned about water pollution since swimming wild. Outdoor swimming inspired them to act, with 68 percent of them increasing their recycling or reusing and 65 percent of them actively engaging in wildlife conservation.

5 Pools come with rules

No bombing, ducking, diving, or running! Keep in that lane and swim at that time. Ensure you swim at a pace that fits into slow, medium, or fast speeds. Lane-rage, kids bumping into you, and someone else's hair wrapping around your fingers can all disrupt your flow. Chlorine and pool chemicals linger on your skin for days, making it dry and itchy. They destroy hair and corrode swimsuits. There are fewer restrictions in wild water and there is space to swim slow or fast. Swims can begin and end where and when you want. Explore beautiful rivers, lay on rocks warmed by the sun, and duck under waterfalls. Sit in scooped-out stones and bathe in the bubbling water rushing between. Feel reeds brush your legs and sink your toes into silt. Swim for long distances with nothing but water behind or ahead, and float belly up to the sky. Sit on riverbanks with hot drinks and cinnamon rolls. Break ice and plunge into water holes. Find sand between your toes. Be naked, exposed, and barefoot. Embrace your feral side, skin your knees, bruise your elbows, and get a muddy bottom. Run, walk, slide, or jump into wild water—it's a freeing place to be.

When submerged, you are just a person, a body, and the water doesn't care where you were born, or what you look like.

6 Anyone can do it

Everyone came from the water, and we can all learn how to swim. No matter who you are, water is a great equalizer. When we are in the water, we are all the same—we are human. We are not what we do for work; it doesn't matter how smart we are, what we have, or what we lack. We are living beings adapting to the environment we swim in. Compared to land-based activities, body type is less relevant. Fat or thin, tall or short, you can achieve in the water. Regardless of our politics or social standing, all of us will gasp at the cold, fear a shark, or enjoy the thrill of the water. When submerged, you are just a person, a body, and the water doesn't care where you were born, or what you look like.

7 It is often free

Unlike gyms, recreation centers, and pools, wild water can cost you nothing. Wild swimming requires very little equipment—in fact if you choose the right spot in the wild, you don't even need a swimsuit! Like any passion or pursuit, there are plenty of opportunities to invest in equipment, books, and tools to enhance your swimming, but one of the most joyful swims you will ever experience is the one that wasn't planned. That maybe happened in just your underwear or naked—air-drying afterward. If you learn enough about the water and your body, you can be spontaneous—there is such freedom that comes from making a dynamic risk assessment in the moment and enjoying a safe swim wildly.

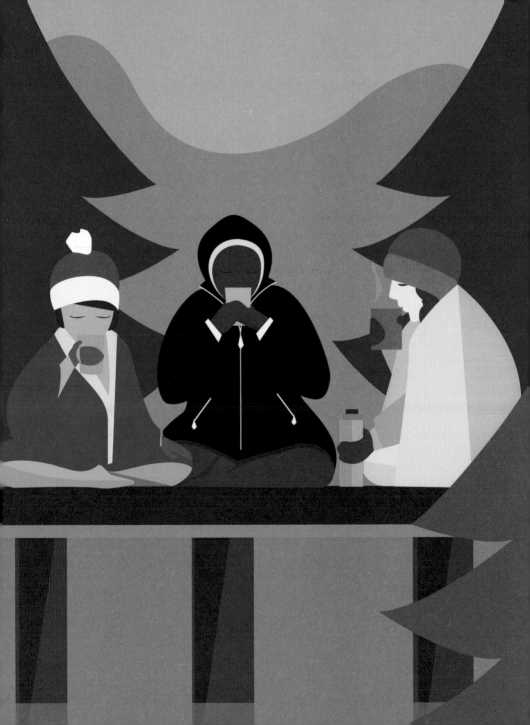

8 It helps with loneliness and isolation

Swimming indoors can be solitary. With your head down and ears submerged, it is just you and the water. By contrast, wild swimming is sociable—it is highly recommended that when in wilder water, you don't swim alone. A riskier activity compared to lifeguarded pools, being with others ensures someone could call for help in an emergency or offer immediate help themselves. But as well as this, wild swimming draws people together. Communities across the world are being established with a shared love of the water. Often informal groups, these tend to start with one swimmer who invites a friend to come along, and then another may witness the swim and ask to join them.

Photographer Ana Elisa Sotelo took to the water in Peru to aid recovery from an injury. She started swimming in the sea for relief from back pain and soon joined Las Truchas—The Trout. The group started as three women, but now there are over 60 members and it's still growing. "From the cold water they emerged transformed: the challenge, discipline, and effort it took to swim helped heal the trauma derived from the pandemic," says Ana. "They set out to arouse this sentiment in other women. In swimming together, they found solidarity, sisterhood, and resilience." Even in the darkest depths of winter, groups can be found huddled together after a cool dip, enjoying hot drinks and chatting.

Communities across the world are being established with a shared love of the water.

9 It increases strength and resilience

Outdoor swimmers often say they feel like they can achieve anything after a cold swim. Early morning dippers claim they have a better outlook on the day if it begins with a dose of wild water. Many have described how being able to tackle cold water sets them up to take on any stresses that enter their life. The physiological response to cold water immersion is similar to how the body reacts to any kind of stress. Dr. Mark Harper, consultant anesthetist at Brighton and Sussex University Hospital and cold-water swimmer, has examined the mental and physical benefits of cold-water immersion. He says, "A cold-water swim can be reorienting. The physical and mental challenges disrupt our sense of time and space, and even of our physical bodies, taking us away from our daily lives. This distance offers an alternative and expanded perspective on our values and issues." A swim can help us escape our thoughts and break anxiety cycles, which can aid problem-solving and improve outlook.

10 It's a sensory experience

Swimming in wild water is a multisensory, full-body experience, unlike many land-based activities. Irish artist Vanessa Daws says, "You can't feel air, but you can feel the water." As well as how swimming can feel when you immerse, wild water offers sweet smells from flower and fauna. Depending on where you swim, it can taste earthy or salty. The sounds of rushing, splashing, or trickling water are in and around your ears. Maybe you can hear birdsong and rustling leaves. Seeing a flash of bright red feathers as a cardinal darts, or the bright yellow of water lily flowers, and the light dancing off the water makes a swim wild. Nothing can help you escape mental chatter and life demands like a swim in wild water. Heart pounding, chest expanding, your body is held. You leave anxiety at the water's edge, wash your worries downstream, and feel naturally high. From the squish underfoot to the sensation of towel fibers on goosebumped skin, wild swimming allows us to feel free.

Nothing can help you escape mental chatter like a swim in wild water.

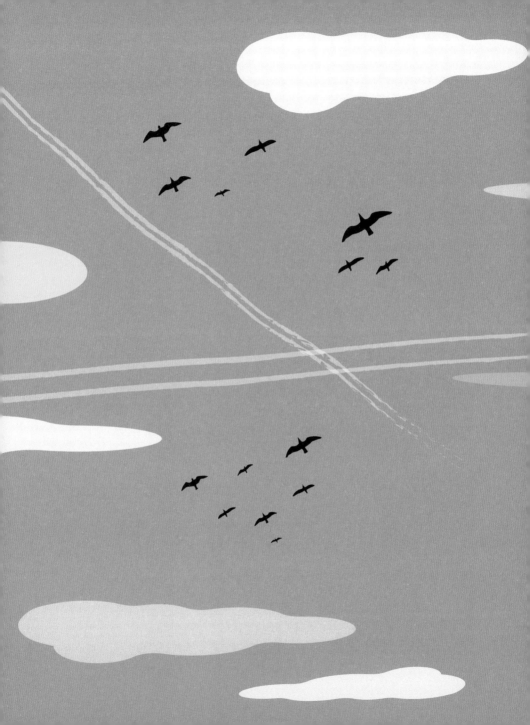

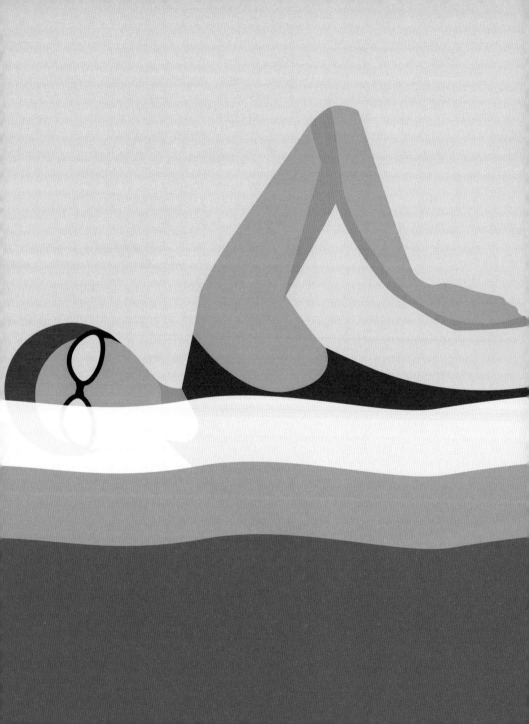

2
CAN
YOU
SWIM?

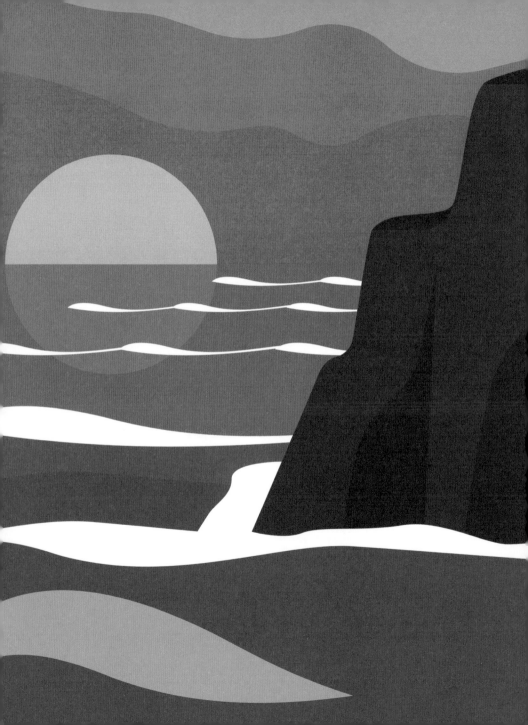

RESPECTING THE WATER

Wild swimming, dipping, and paddling can seem like a simple, relaxed way to enjoy the water without any particular swimming prowess. But it's essential you know how to swim before you enter wild water.

For a long time, I ignorantly believed that most people learned to swim at a young age. I did when I was four years old and I have never feared the water. I remember very early on in my wild river swimming encouraging a non-swimmer to give it a try. We were in a beautiful river pool under a series of falls and there were plenty of places to put your feet down. It was so unimaginable to me that someone couldn't even float around safely in the water that it seemed friendly to encourage them to join in. Luckily a more experienced wild swimmer put me in my place and told the person to stay safely on land. I felt scolded and embarrassed, but I look back with gratitude. While I had positive intentions, wanting to share the joy of the water, I had no real idea what I was offering. I didn't know how that person would respond to the cold, rushing, wild water and I had no clue how to support or save them if needed.

Today, I am better skilled at supporting new swimmers. I can teach, coach, and even rescue if needed. I have witnessed the very real fear of the water when trying to teach or coach a new swimmer, I understand how quickly someone can lose their life in the water, and I have felt the grip and discomfort of a non-swimmer while attempting to teach. One of the biggest issues in the water is panic, so it's important to know what to expect. The following pages will help you safely prepare for your wild swim.

When was your last swim?

Maybe, like me, you were lucky enough to be taught to swim at a young age. Since learning, you may have dipped in and out of leisure pools, paddled and swam at the beach while on vacation, or swam a few lengths as a cool-down after the gym. But ask yourself, when was the last time you went for a real swim? When you swam 25 meters or further without putting your feet down?

Lots of people assume that because they are in good health, are reasonably fit, and can swim, they will be able to swim confidently in open water. But some people can have incredible land fitness and struggle in the water. Swimming is a skill, and doing it outside demands more. Swimming requires technique to breathe and skill to keep your head above water long enough to do so. If you can't float, tread water, or be out of your depth in a calm and relaxed manner, you don't have the basic skills for a wild swim. If you can't swim, learn. Find a local pool and ask them about swimming lessons. Many adults can't swim and there is no shame in that. If you can swim, but it has been a while, get to the pool. Swim some lengths without putting your feet down. See how you feel—exhausted? Breathless? Maybe you need to work on your technique (see pages 135–145).

The best way to stay safe in open water is to become swim fit.

Are you swim fit?

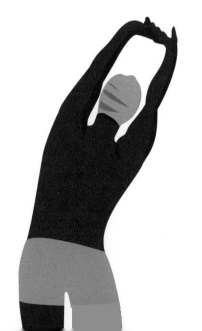

Swimming is a physical activity that requires fitness, strength, flexibility, and coordination. When wild swimming you need all this, as well as courage, stamina, and skills that aid swimming in outdoor conditions (see pages 135–145). As a beginner in wild water, it is good to consider some basics. Swimming is rhythmic, and being comfortable in the water is key. It is good to think about how strong a swimmer you are and how you can keep yourself safe. If needed, could you swim against a current? Would you be able to swim through or over waves? Could you keep yourself calm and swim through weeds and past wildlife? The best way to stay safe in open water is to become swim fit. This means being able to move effortlessly in the water without tiring. Many people complain about exhausting themselves or running out of breath when swimming, but this can indicate poor technique. It is common for people to hold their breath too much, kick too hard, and splash around exerting lots of energy while not getting very far. The very best way to swim wild is calmly, consistently, and strongly (see pages 135–145 for more on swimming technique).

Pool practice

Swimming pools are fantastic places to learn to swim, work on technique, establish skill, gain confidence, and build stamina. The more time you can spend in the water, learning and understanding your body in a safe environment, the better.

Often the biggest challenge with pool swimming is other people. Finding your place in the pool for practice at a comfortable pace can be hard. Generally, public recreation centers offer lane-swimming sessions throughout the day. Try different times to figure out what type of swimmers are swimming at your local pool and when. You don't want to be heading to the pool during a busy family session; conversely, often the last lane session of the day is empty, so you can make the most of your time in the water.

It might seem obvious, but wild swimming is very different than swimming in a pool. Many don't consider what it is like to swim without being able to see the bottom, which isn't guaranteed in wild water. Add the cooler water temperature, weeds, wildlife, weather, currents, tides, and waves and consider how confident you feel about swimming wild.

Use the pool to practice swimming in deep water without putting your feet down. Start with a 30-minute swim session and try to do a variety of different swim strokes. See how many lengths you can swim without stopping, building up your stamina. A pool is great for learning to float, tread water, and swim distance. An outdoor swimming pool is a good transition from a pool into open water. It allows you to experience colder water while still swimming in a man-made structure.

Learning to float

Developing the ability to float can unlock swimming skills and help overcome fear of the water. Floating also improves balance and control of the body.

Being able to float comfortably on your back in the wild is a wonderful experience, as well as a simple lifesaving skill. I love being able to roll onto my back and watch the clouds pass, or float under a tree canopy. Being rocked gently by the ocean while floating or taken downstream on a wide, deep river is transformative. As well as a fantastic feeling, floating on our backs enables our faces to be out of the water, giving us time to breathe and calm ourselves. We can also shout for help if needed.

Floating is hard if you are nervous or afraid, so practice in a pool to find a sense of ease. The human body is naturally buoyant, our lungs full of air, so in theory everyone can float.

Being able to float comfortably on your back in the wild is a wonderful experience, as well as a simple lifesaving skill.

Tips

— Practice with a friend—get them to hold your head and/or shoulders until you're in position and then gently let go once you're relaxed

— When practicing, start within your depth, with your feet on the floor. But once you have mastered the move, you can transition into a star float from a relaxed position when swimming out of your depth

— Use a pool noodle—a long foam float—under the shoulders and/or head to practice the position

— Imagine someone tying string to your belly button and pulling it up

— Challenge yourself to float for 5, 10, 15... 60 seconds

— Once you are comfortable in the pool, take it outside

How to float

Let's start with a star float—this is when your body floats on the surface of the water with arms and legs extended and apart, opened into an X-shape. This will stabilize your body and stop you from rolling over. Make as big a shape as possible to cover the greatest surface area. Once you're in position, relax. The more tense you are in your body the more you will roll up and sink.

1 Start in a relaxed upright position, with your shoulders under the water and legs directly beneath your body.

2 Take a deep breath and gently lean backward into the water, until your ears are submerged under the water and your eyes are looking up to the sky.

3 As your body and legs automatically rise, push your tummy up and extend your legs and arms into an X-shape.

Once you're in position, ensure your neck is long and extended, your tummy and hips are pushed up, and your arms and legs are straight. You should be looking up toward the sky with both your ears submerged. In this position you should be able to regulate your breathing.

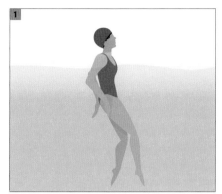

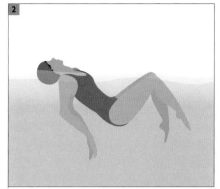

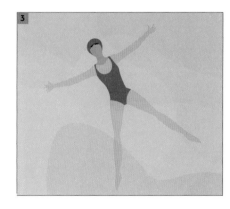

How to tread water

Treading water enables you to maintain an upright position, keeping you afloat while staying in the same place. Arms should be working along with your legs to keep the body in a vertical position. The following leg and arm techniques encourage you to move in a way that doesn't propel you but keeps you afloat with minimal effort. Practice in the pool, within your depth first.

Leg techniques

Use any of these techniques in conjunction with your chosen arm action (see page 35).

Egg beater

This is an alternating breaststroke kick and is the most efficient method to use.

1 Start in an upright position with your shoulders clear of the water.

2 Bend each leg as in a frog kick, one at a time, alternating legs. The heel of your bent leg should be toward your bottom with your knee pointing outward.

3 With a flexed foot, push the water downward and outward as if you are stamping. In this continuous motion your hips should be flexibly moving your legs in an almost circular action. As one leg kicks down, the other should be rising up.

EGG BEATER

Breaststroke kick

1 Start in an upright position with your shoulders clear of the water.

2 Bend both legs at the same time into a frog kick position, heels toward your bottom and knees pointing outward. Feet should be flexed to push the water downward.

3 Push your legs around and down until they are vertical in the water.

4 Bring your legs around and back up into the frog kick position before pushing down again. Both legs should move together, mirroring each other.

Crawl kick

1 Start in an upright position with your shoulders clear of the water.

2 With your legs in a vertical position, continuously kick your feet backward and forward using small, fast movements.

Bicycle kick

1 Start in an upright position with your shoulders clear of the water.

2 Move your legs in a continuous circular motion as if you are pedaling on a bike, one knee up and then the other. Picture your legs pushing down on imaginary pedals, forcing the water downward.

Scissor kick

1 Start in an upright position with your shoulders clear of the water.

2 Split your legs apart, one leg in front of you and one behind.

3 Then bring them together, keeping the knees soft.

4 Once they have come together, split them apart again, taking the same leg out in front. Repeat this continual motion—imagine a pair of scissors and how the blades move together and then apart. This leg action creates a bobbing movement in the water, which pushes your body upward.

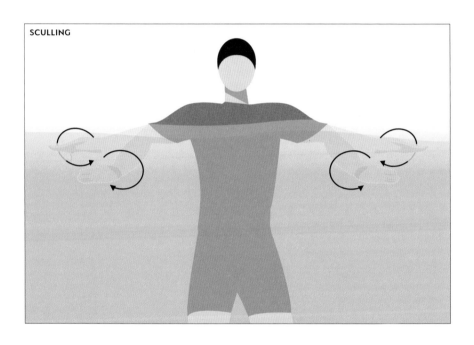

SCULLING

Arm techniques

Use any of these techniques in conjunction with your chosen leg action (see pages 32–33).

Sculling

1 Start in an upright position with your shoulders clear of the water.

2 Extend your arms out sideways, on either side of your body, and let them float just below the surface, with your elbows slightly bent and palms facing down. Move your hands in toward your body and then out away from the sides of your body, using the wrists for movement. Keep your fingers together and cup the water, moving it from side to side. You can imagine making a figure-of-eight shape with your hands. Do this continuously with both hands, keeping them in line with the forearms.

Breaststroke action

This is a breaststroke motion used in a supporting movement, rather than for propulsion.

1 Start in an upright position with your shoulders clear of the water.

2 Move the arms like you would in swimming the breaststroke, extending them in front of you, with hands together, then separating your arms outward to make a circular shape.

3 Bring the hands back to the chest, but don't bring them completely together, and remain in an upright position so that you stay in one place rather than move forward.

4 Then once again extend your arms and circle them outward. Continue this breaststroke motion.

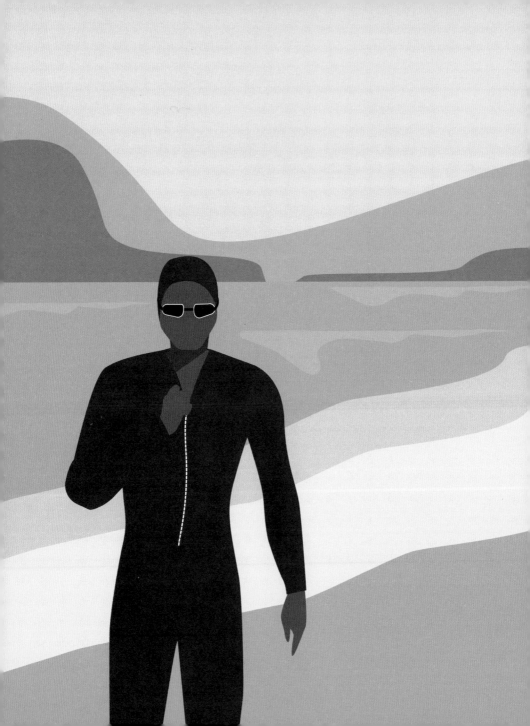

3

WHAT

TO

WEAR

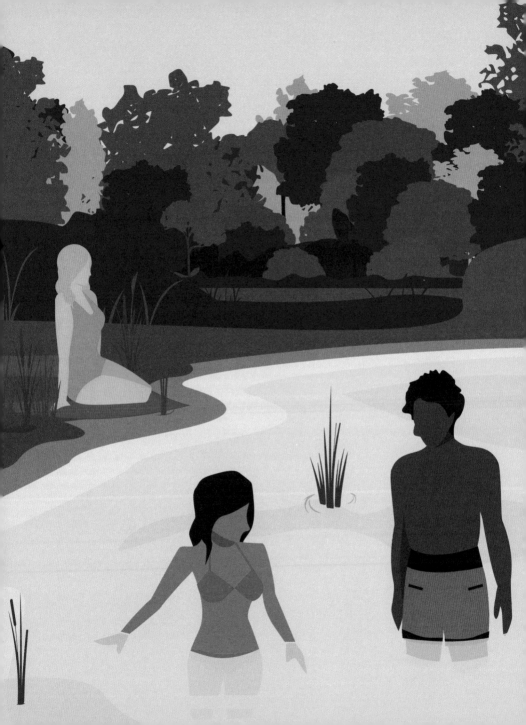

SELECTING YOUR SWIMWEAR

One of the best things about wild swimming is the need for very little equipment. Find a spot remote enough and you don't even need a swimsuit. The best thing to wear when swimming is something that supports you in the way you want and is comfortable. Don't feel awkward wearing a wetsuit when others are not. Equally, if you love a bikini, wear it!

There is a lot of commentary about swimwear, particularly for women. When people started swimming, we were all naked. It will be no surprise that swimwear was introduced to stop peeping men and to "save" women from being exposed to naked males. Swimwear was introduced in the 1700s for both men and women, although the thin cloth often left little to the imagination when wet. Throughout the centuries many different materials and styles of swimwear have been worn. In the past, you could have been banned from a pool for having the wrong kind of swimsuit, and in the 1900s men patrolled American beaches measuring the lengths of ladies' swimsuits to ensure they were not too short. Today, luckily, we have more freedom and choice than ever. The biggest challenge people face when buying swimwear is finding something suitable for their body shape and feeling confident enough to wear it. Swimwear is the closest piece of clothing to underwear and nudity, so it can come with added anxiety.

Wetsuits, swimsuits, shorts, jammers, pants, bikinis, burkinis, leggings, rash guards, or nothing—they all have their benefits. As well as style and type, it is also worth considering the fabric, and features like zippers and ties.

Before you choose what to wear, consider the type of swimming you are going to do. If you are heading to the water for a quick dip, you might choose something very different than you would for a longer swim. Also consider the season and conditions. If I am plunging in and out of waterfalls, I might wear a different swimsuit than one I'd wear swimming in a flat, calm sea.

Swimwear can vary greatly in price, so you can spend as much or as little as you're comfortable with. As with any fitness clothing, find the right fit. If you're in the position to, don't be afraid to invest in your swimwear—it may make you feel more comfortable and could even improve your swimming.

You should choose what to wear based on your own needs and comfort.

Swimsuits and bikinis

There are thousands of different types of one-piece swimsuits and bikinis. Different colors and patterns are personal choice, but their design and function are worth thinking about for your needs. You want your swimwear to be snug, but not tight. It should feel like a second skin, but not leave red marks when you take it off. If it's too loose it will fight with the water, causing drag and discomfort.

Straps

Thicker straps will be more supportive of bigger busts. Thin straps that cross over across the back, or racerback style, can give greater comfort and movement around the shoulders. Consider the fabric and feel of strapping around your armpit to avoid chafing.

Neckline

A higher neckline at the front will reduce drag and scooping up water as you swim. Swimwear that covers your back to the neck can feel warmer in cooler water and windy conditions.

Zippers and ties

Zippers make it easier to get in and out of your suit, but make sure they are strong at the front so that they don't zip down while swimming. Zippers at the back can be uncomfortable if you are wearing a wetsuit over the top. Side ties tend to be fussy, unsupportive, and mostly decorative, but ties at the front of bikini bottoms can be good to tighten and secure.

Bust support

Lots of swimwear comes with adjustable straps for better bust support. There are also suits that have invisible breast panels, but they are not as sculpting as wired or more structured swimwear. Padded cups tend to soak up water and drag when swimming. Regardless of shape or size, your chest should be supported but not squashed by your swimsuit. If your breasts move too much, it can cause chafing on the nipples and under the arms. Some brands will adapt a suit with a pocket if you have had breast cancer and use a prosthetic.

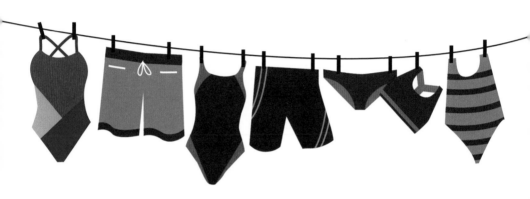

High or low leg cut

Whether you go for a high-cut or low-cut leg is mostly your personal choice, but a high-cut leg offers greater freedom of movement in the water. The fabric shouldn't cut into the skin and again should feel comfortable to avoid chafing.

Fabric

A lot of swimwear brands now use eco fibers that are made from recycled plastics. This makes your suit more environmentally friendly, plus this type of fabric is more resistant to chlorine and salt water. When swimming outside, make sure your swimwear offers UV protection.

Board shorts, briefs, trunks, and jammers

While some swimmers prefer the modesty of baggier shorts, perfect for dipping, others may opt for more streamlined swimwear to improve their swimming speed.

Board shorts

Made from lightweight materials, board shorts are a popular choice for leisure swimming. They can be a modest and comfortable choice.

Briefs or trunks

Some people find tighter-fitting trunks or briefs easier to swim in than baggy shorts, which can slow you down. Trunks or briefs made famous by Speedo are often associated with more competitive swimming but are favored by many outdoor swimmers.

Jammers

Jammers are a longer, snug-fitting style that comes down to the knee. They can offer the advantages of briefs, but with a little more modesty.

Buoyancy shorts

If your legs feel heavy in the water and you struggle to float, buoyancy shorts could be a great choice. They have panels in the backs of the legs and bottom to help lift and give a more horizontal position in the water.

Tips

~ Board shorts are better the shorter they are. They offer modesty but can be uncomfortable when wet. Avoid below-the-knee length, which can restrict leg-kick movement. Shorts will crumple under a wetsuit and may be uncomfortable.

~ Briefs or trunks can feel revealing but offer less drag and chafing, and more freedom of movement in the water. They are also better under a wetsuit.

Modest swimwear

Wild water welcomes everyone, and the most important thing is that a swimmer be comfortable, and feel confident and safe. You may opt for modest swimwear for cultural, religious, health, or personal reasons, seeking something that covers your arms and legs—and that is safe to swim in and feels comfortable. Big brands have developed swim hijabs complete with swim leggings and long-sleeved tops, but now independent brands are coming to market offering more stylish, fun, and sustainable choices. The biggest challenge with modest swimwear is that it can pull and drag more than standard suits.

Tips

— Try to avoid suits with too much fabric—while it might look good, it can wrap around you and make it harder to swim

— Ensure the fabric is durable and light enough to get wet for swimming

— Snug swim leggings with a looser tunic will be better for swimming

The most important thing is that a swimmer be comfortable, and feel confident and safe.

Wetsuits

Wetsuits are a useful yet much debated piece of equipment for outdoor swimmers. They are a fairly recent phenomenon, only invented in the 1950s with outdoor swimming–specific wetsuits being introduced in the 1980s. Open-water swimming has a long tradition of participants not wearing wetsuits—swimmers either learned how to adapt to cold water or they didn't swim at all. Many marathon swimming events across the world and great swims like the English Channel still don't allow wetsuit swims to be recognized as a genuine crossing.

A "skins" swimmer is someone who swims without a wetsuit, in a standard swimsuit, goggles, and swim cap. There is often debate around wearing a wetsuit versus "skins" swimming, and purists will tell you that wild swimming is not done in a wetsuit. But I say, if you feel safe and comfortable swimming in a wetsuit, then you should. Wild swimming isn't for medals and glory, it is for joy!

A wetsuit is ultimately designed to provide thermal protection when you are wet. Not to be confused with a dry suit, a wetsuit allows water to enter the suit, while a dry suit prevents water from entering. Wetsuits are usually made from neoprene, and designed for different uses and temperatures. They work by letting water into the suit, thus creating a thin layer of water between the rubbery fabric and the skin, which then heats up and insulates the swimmer.

Traditionally wetsuits were used for diving, surfing, and above-water sports. When triathlon evolved—a sporting event that consists of an open-water swim, a bike ride, and a run—athletes used wetsuits for the swim to keep them warm, but it also enabled them to swim faster. Another benefit of a wetsuit is that they make you more buoyant in the water, which can aid swimming and increase your speed. As outdoor swimming became fashionable again, many triathlon organizers started offering swim-only events and followed triathlon rules that allow wetsuits rather than requiring traditional "skins" swimming, which meant that, for a while, wetsuits were in vogue and it was more unusual to swim "skins." But recently, with the rise in wild, cold, outdoor swimming for joyful leisure purposes and mental health, more and more swimmers swim "skins."

A wetsuit tends to be a bigger investment than a swimsuit, but now more than ever there is a greater variety of style and price points. Because of the wide choice, it can be confusing to know what you might need and daunting to buy one. Different styles and thickness can make it baffling to new outdoor swimmers, so wherever you choose to purchase your wetsuit, do some research and ask questions.

Advantages

— Will keep you warmer and enable longer swims

— Increases buoyancy

— Can be designed to increase swim speed

— Supports swimmers year-round in cooler temperatures

Disadvantages

— Additional cost

— Another thing to carry

— Difficult to get on and off

— Removes the sensory experience of water

— Can cause chafing and discomfort around the neck

— Many wetsuits are designed for crawl and aren't suitable for breaststroke

A wetsuit should feel tight when you first put it on, but not so much you can't move your arms!

Things to consider

→ The more expensive a suit, the more design features for speed. An expensive suit is often more technical and thinner, and will give greater flexibility. Cheaper, mid-range suits will offer more warmth and are harder wearing.

→ Think about how often you plan to swim and what sort of swims you are doing. If you are swimming two or three times a week and covering some distance, it will be worth spending a little more than if you are only indulging in occasional dips.

→ Ensure it fits well. Too tight and it will limit movement and breathing. Too loose and it will fill with water, cancel the thermal benefits, and make it harder to swim.

→ Look at the manufacturer's size guide and measure yourself to choose the best fit. It should feel tight when you first put it on, but not so much you can't move your arms!

→ Swimming wetsuits were developed for events and racing, so don't always suit a more casual breaststroke swimmer. However, brands have responded to the demand of leisure swimmers and now offer wetsuits more suitable for breaststroke swimming. The paneling is different, which means the legs are not as buoyant as with other suits.

→ Consider renting, borrowing, or buying second-hand to decide whether a wetsuit is for you. They do feel different to swim in. Many venues offer wetsuit rental, which is a good way to try before you buy, and lots of brands have discounts and offers at the end of the summer season.

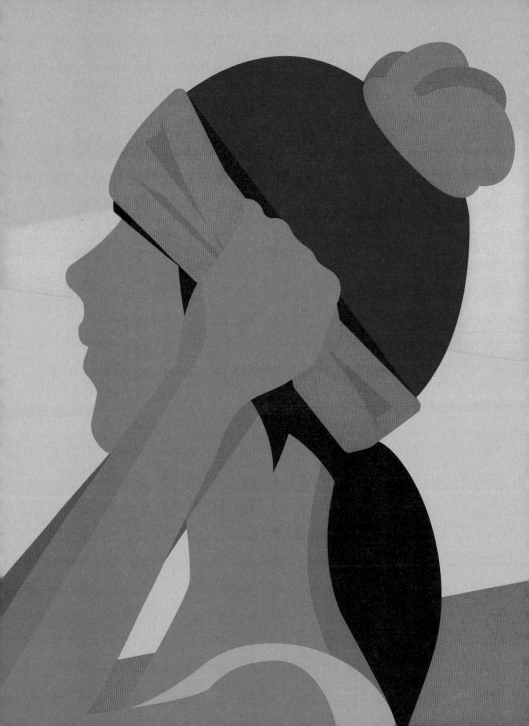

4

SWIM GEAR

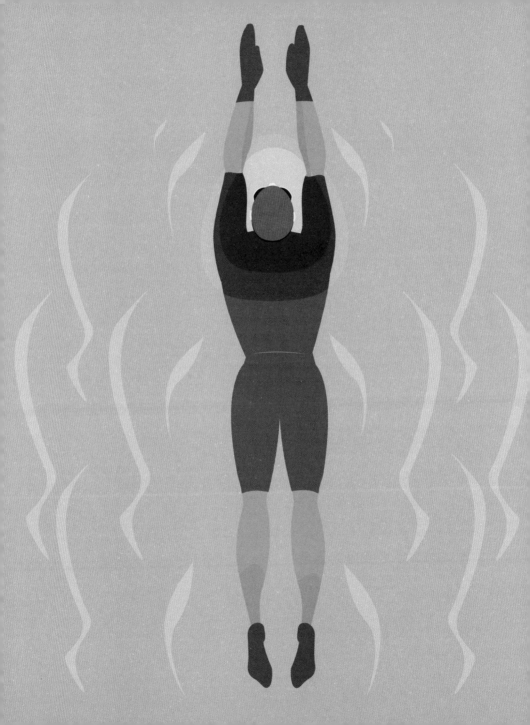

CHOOSING YOUR GEAR

Wild swimming, at its best, is spontaneous and requires very little equipment. But if you want to become a regular outdoor swimmer, a bit of gear can aid, improve, and make your swimming safer. As with any leisure pursuit, you could spend a lot of money on gear, gadgets, and tools that promise to make your swimming better in any number of ways, but just a few simple extras could be all you need. Once you have sorted out what you are going to wear on your body, the next two items, which are not essential but are the minimum when it comes to swimming gear, are a swim cap and a pair of goggles. Then depending on where you are swimming, how far, or for how long, there are other pieces of additional gear that could help your swimming. The following pages will guide you through the most useful gear.

Swim caps and knit hats

Swimming caps are not always a favorite—we may have bad memories of rubber hats pulling at our heads as kids when learning to swim, but they have come a long way since their invention in the early twentieth century.

Choosing a swim cap

Shop around and you will discover there is a huge variety of sizing, materials, and functions. Fit is all-important. If it is too tight or small, it can come off during your swim or give you a tension headache. There are three main types of material used for swim caps—latex, silicone, and neoprene—although you can still get ahold of vintage rubber hats and new cotton or fabric hats.

LATEX Cheaper, thinner, and stretches better. Tears easily.

SILICONE Softer, thicker, and hard-wearing. A firm favorite.

NEOPRENE Ideal for cold water, warmest choice. Only to be used in the cold.

Advantages

— Reduces heat loss through the head and helps with brain freeze in colder water

— Brightly colored hats are safer, increasing your visibility in the water

— They can keep hair out of your face and protect your hair from salt

— Caps can identify a team, group, or level of ability

— Can be useful for storing medication, car keys, or feeding gels in events

Shop around for swim caps and you will discover that there is a huge variety of sizing, materials, and functions.

RUBBER Old-fashioned, thick, but often fun designs.

COTTON/NYLON FABRIC Better for children as easy to get on and off.

Some of the leading swim brands offer different-sized swimming caps. SOUL CAP is a FINA (the international swimming federation) approved brand and a designer of swim hats for big hair. They offer a range of sizes and colors, great for thick, curly, long, or afro hair.

Knit hats

Swimmers may swap their cap for a knit hat in cooler months, opting to keep their head out of the water entirely to avoid that brain-freeze feeling. In windy, cold temperatures, a bobble hat can help keep you warm for a little longer. Natural fibers like wool are best for both practical and environmental reasons—a wool hat can keep you warm even if it gets wet, and if any fibers end up in the water, it's better that they be natural.

Earplugs

Goggles

I never swim without earplugs. It's mainly because I hate the feathery feeling of water in my ears when I get out, but when you swim a lot, you are at risk for infection. And if you swim frequently in cold water without earplugs, you are at risk for swimmer's ear (see page 109). Again, there are lots of different options out there and cheap ways to prevent water from entering the ear canal; here are three main types of earplugs:

PLASTIC AND SILICONE MIX Soft silicone that fits inside the ear, with a plastic wing for inserting and taking out. Best for still being able to hear and for a small ear canal.

SILICONE ERGONOMICALLY SHAPED Extra protection for the outer ear, easy to insert and remove.

SOFT MOLDABLE SILICONE Mold to the shape of your ear, but harder to hear when wearing them.

The oldest reference to anything like goggles is in the fourteenth century, but goggles as we know them today were first developed in the early twentieth century. Thomas Burgess, the second person to swim across the English Channel, used a pair of motorcycle goggles in 1911 to help him tackle the chop and swell of the sea. In 1926, when Gertrude Ederle became the first woman to swim across the English Channel, she used a similar goggle to Burgess' but made hers waterproof using a paraffin seal. While there were various patents submitted for eye protection and goggle-like designs, the first commercial goggles were not sold until the 1960s. Today, there are thousands of brands and designs available.

The main use of goggles is to keep water out of your eyes so that you can see where you are going. As a swimming teacher, when I first work with new swimmers, many of them have never worn or thought to use goggles.

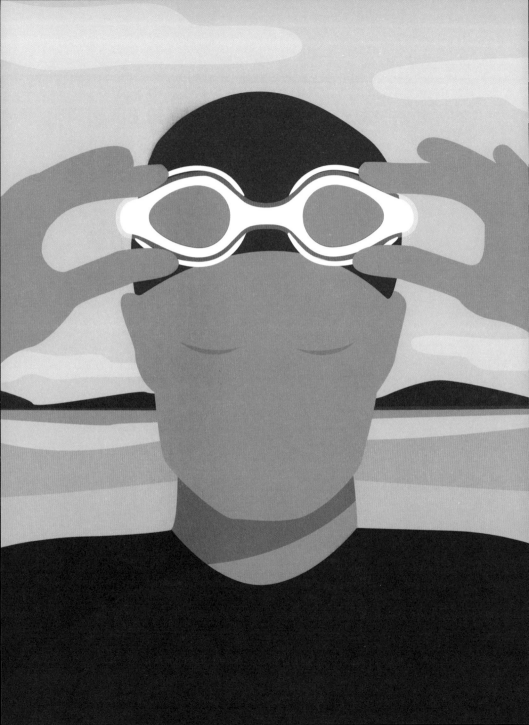

Sea swimming, clear rivers, and freshwater lakes can offer an underwater playground.

While you may have no intention of putting your head in the water, especially outside, a pair of goggles can protect your eyes from chlorine, salt water, and dirt. Even a splash can render you temporarily blind without goggles. While there is generally no real harm in getting water in your eyes, a pair of goggles can make it easier for you to get your face in the water, which results in a better swim position where you expend less energy and can swim farther or for longer.

There's an underwater world to explore, too. While some people may prefer not to see what's beneath, and a lot of the time you can't see much at all, there are plenty of swimming spots that are worthy of goggles. Sea swimming, clear rivers, and freshwater lakes can offer an underwater playground. I have collected my favorite shells and sea treasures when swimming. My home is full of pebbles, smoothed glass, shells, and even rusty metal I have discovered while exploring the world in the water. I would have missed the turtle I was swimming with off the Turkish coast if I hadn't had my goggles on, and who can argue that it isn't better to see where you are going?

Choosing goggles

It's hard to recommend goggles; there are so many choices and so many different face shapes and preferences. The only real way to find out what suits you is to try some out. At a minimum you need your goggles to be watertight and comfortable—not too tight around your eye sockets. They also need a suitable lens; a clear lens is better for indoor swimming, and a tinted lens is great for bright, sunny days outside.

SMALL LENSES are popular for competitive and pool swimming. They should fit comfortably into the eye socket and often have an adjustable nose bridge.

OPEN-WATER GOGGLES have larger lenses and tend to sit on the bone around the eye, rather than in the socket. They enable a wider field of vision and also have more lens varieties—tinted, mirrored, and polarized, for example.

MASK-STYLE GOGGLES sit on the cheekbones and provide extra face coverage. These can help tackle the cold and offer a big field of vision. They don't cover the nose like diving masks.

Prescription goggles

If you wear glasses, you have a few options. It's not advisable to wear contact lenses under goggles due to the risk of infection if water gets in your eyes. If your prescription isn't that strong, you could muddle along with just regular goggles. You can buy off-the-shelf prescription goggles for approximate correction, or you can get custom prescription lens goggles.

Tips

— All goggles have adjustable straps to fit your head and face shape, so use them to fit the goggles properly. A good pair should stay put without leaving hard rings around your eyes after swimming.

— Read the product description and manufacturer's guidance when buying to ensure your goggles will suit your swimming style and face shape.

— If you're spending money on a decent pair of goggles, or prescription goggles, take good care of them. Ensure they are rinsed off in fresh water and leave them to air-dry after swimming. Keep them in a case to prevent scratches and scuffs.

— Once you find a pair you like, consider buying a spare pair and a couple of lens varieties: clear for gray, dark days and tinted for sunny swims.

— All goggles now come with anti-fog protection on interior lenses, but after time the effect can wear off. Saliva is the simplest and safest way to combat foggy goggles, so licking the inside of your lenses can help.

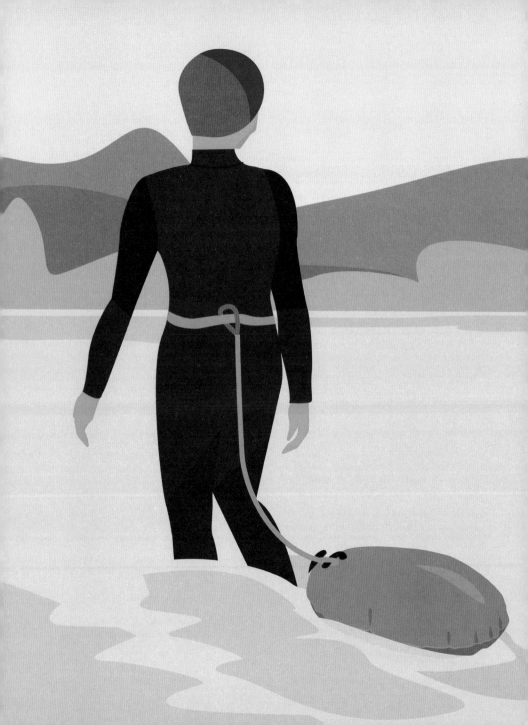

Tow floats

A tow float is an inflated, brightly colored device that is tethered to a swimmer, enabling them to be more easily seen by other water users and from land. While not a lifesaving device, they are designed to keep you safer in the water and offer some buoyancy.

Tow floats have gone from being a geeky aid to a must-have accessory. A modern invention, created in response to the rise of open-water swimming in the UK, they are now used worldwide. Their primary purpose is to increase visibility in the water, but there are many variations that offer other functions.

One of the most useful developments of the tow float is that they can provide a way to carry anything from clothes, a towel, water, medicines, and snacks to valuable items like a mobile phone and your car keys. They also enable you to swim from one place to another as there is no need to leave your belongings behind. Plus you can use your phone to call for help if needed.

They are simple to use, and all types generally come with a waist strap, a line to connect to the float, and the float itself. You simply inflate it and strap it to you, or fill it with stuff and then inflate it before strapping it to your body. As you swim, the tow float is pulled behind you. You can use it to rest on if needed, and it has little impact on your swimming.

Since the invention of tow floats there have been innovations and new ideas based on the simple design. Bigger floating devices have been developed, which mean you can now go on more adventurous swims and trips, carrying bulkier items like tents, so you can combine your wild swim with camping.

Shoes, socks, and gloves

When I take first-time wild swimmers out in the water, one of the most common questions is, "What should I wear on my feet?" As with swimsuits, hats, and goggles it largely comes down to personal preference and where you plan to swim. I have a vague personal rule that if I am swimming in a river, somewhere with rocks and shingle, or in an undiscovered place for me I will wear something on my feet to protect them from jabbing, piercing, and injuries. I love the feel of the water, and something on my hands and feet diminishes that, but at times I have been so grateful to have them covered.

Feet

Most people have soft, supple skin on the bottom of their feet, making walking or standing on rocks or shingle uncomfortable, and it is easily cut, which puts us at risk for infection. As well as natural hazards like sharp stones and rock, there are man-made items that are often found near water—like fishing hooks or broken glass. It is a sad fact that humans leave things behind when visiting beautiful places like beaches and riverbanks, so we need to take care.

Choosing footwear

Protecting our feet can impact our swimming, so finding something suitable is important. As wild swimming has boomed, so have the foot-care options.

NOTHING Bare feet on squishy mud, soft clay, or sand brings joy. There is real pleasure in fully embracing the feral state of going barefoot. Do a visual risk assessment before you take your shoes off, though.

A FLIP-FLOP, SLIDER, CROC, OR SHOWER SHOE They are cheap, waterproof, and can protect your feet while walking toward the water's edge. Easy to get on and off as you enter and get out of the water.

AN OLD PAIR OF SOCKS I often recommend these for beginners if they want to protect their feet but don't want to invest too much. While sharp items might still pierce through the fabric, a thick pair of socks can give some protection. They do get heavy and flappy when wet, but for dipping can be enough.

A WATER SHOE There are many different types and price ranges. Generally they have a rubber sole and netted fabric to help water drain away. Cheaper versions can be bought at supermarkets or beach shops, often worn for paddling and play, but are useless for swimming.

A SWIMMING SHOE They have a rubber sole and fit snugly to ensure they don't fill with water. My favorite kind separates the toes like gloves and the sole is thin and flexible.

NEOPRENE SOCKS These are great for swimming in cold water. Our feet don't have much fat on them to keep them warm, so they cool quickly and can hurt in the cold. They can also numb and then you can't feel what you are

Tips

— Ensure a tight, snug fit so that the socks or shoes don't fill with water

— Make sure the sole is thick, but flexible so you can swim, and has good grip for walking or stepping out of the water

— A strap that fastens around the foot or ankle often stops them from slipping off or filling with water

stepping on. Neoprene socks allow your feet to stay warm, and most are designed with a thicker sole that protects your feet.

Hands

Not many wild swimmers wear gloves. They are mostly used by those swimming in cold water. If you have a health condition like arthritis (pain and inflammation in joints) or Reynaud's syndrome (blood circulation issues), gloves can reduce symptoms and discomfort. Like our toes and feet, hands and fingers have very little fat on them, so they are more prone to the cold. They will cool quicker, numb, and can get very painful.

Choosing gloves

Neoprene gloves can make a huge difference, keeping hands warmer for longer and preventing numbing, which when getting dressed is useful for zippers and buttons. There are lots of brands that offer neoprene gloves—the most important thing is that they fit. Too big and they will fill with water, becoming heavy and hard to swim in. Too tight and you will find them difficult to get on and off.

Tips

— Measure your hands and use the size guides when buying gloves

— Wrist straps on gloves can be useful, preventing them from coming off or filling with water

Neoprene gloves can make a huge difference.

Towels and robes

You don't really need much more than a towel when it comes to drying off and changing, especially in warm and calm conditions. Changing on beaches, riverbanks, or in any wild place becomes normal and routine the more you do it. You will find your own ways to dry and change quickly when needed.

The best thing to do after an outdoor swim is to remove wet items, dry off, and get dressed. Your body continues to cool when out of the water, even on a warm day, so unless you are swimming in a heatwave it's worth drying off properly. It doesn't really matter what kind of towel you have, but microfiber towels dry quicker, roll up smaller, and are light for adventure swims. Turkish-style hammam towels are similar. Or I love nothing more than a giant beach towel for laying on after a swim when conditions are right.

Robes made from toweling or microfiber are great for throwing on after a swim

and changing under. They were designed to help us change with some modesty while drying us at the same time. A changing robe is bigger with a fleece or toweling lining and a weatherproof outer. They are also big enough to change under and will protect you from the elements as you change. Robes have developed into a bit of a cult product, with celebrities seen walking dogs and supermarket shopping in them. They can be expensive and cumbersome, so they are not for everyone or every kind of swim. They are great in winter or poor weather, but can be too big to carry on adventure swims and too hot for summer dips.

Often, I see people throw on a dry robe in their swimsuit and that's that, they are heading home. But this will mean that the inner robe will now be wet, so their body will still be cooling. A robe can be useful if you dry off a little first and then get changed under it. That way you will get warmer more quickly and be protected from the weather as you dress.

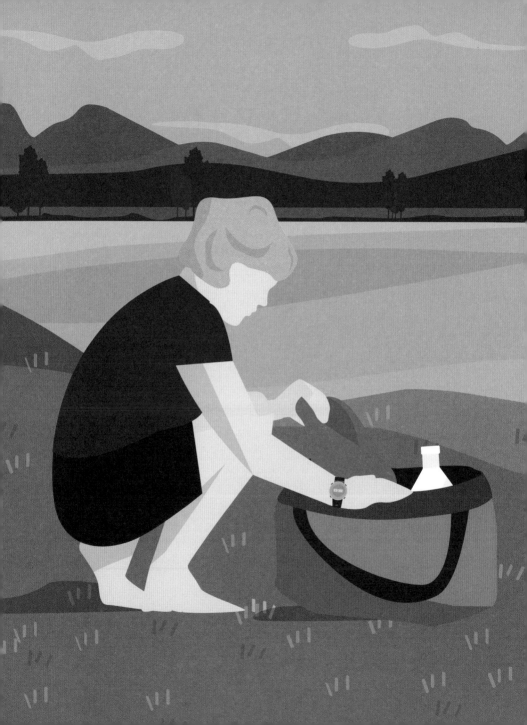

Gadgets and other equipment

Of course, the list of gear could go on and on. There are lots of gadgets, training devices, things to wear, and gear you can take on your swim. You can buy everything from a pop-up changing room to goggles that indicate when you are swimming in a straight line. I stand by my statement that the best wild swims are spontaneous and feral. But here are some things I often take on a swim or keep in my bag.

A small, basic first-aid kit

I cut and scrape myself, and get stung, more than I should. It's always useful to have for yourself and others.

Waterproof watch

Essential for sea swimming to know what time it is for tide movement, but also great to know how long you have been in the water in winter. Some watches also track distance and speed.

Waterproof camera

I love to capture the beauty and joy of a swim, from wildlife to pals leaping in.

Whistle

A cheap and simple safety device. Good for swimming in large stretches of open water, difficult weather, and night swimming. Blowing on it can get the attention of other swimmers, alert someone on land to assist you, and help someone locate you in the water.

Changing mat

This could be an old towel or plastic bag to stand on. It prevents everything from getting wet and dirty while you are changing.

Waterproof lights

If swimming at night or in low-light conditions, I recommend not straying too far from land. It is also worth lighting the area where you plan to get in and out of the water. Camping lights are useful here. You can also buy adventure lights that are waterproof, durable, and super bright. These are made with clips that can be attached to goggle straps, tow floats, or swimsuit straps, making you visible in the water.

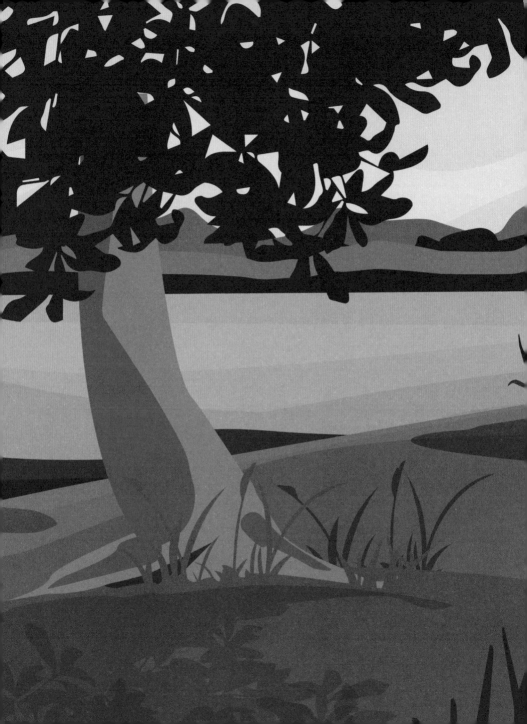

5

WHERE TO SWIM

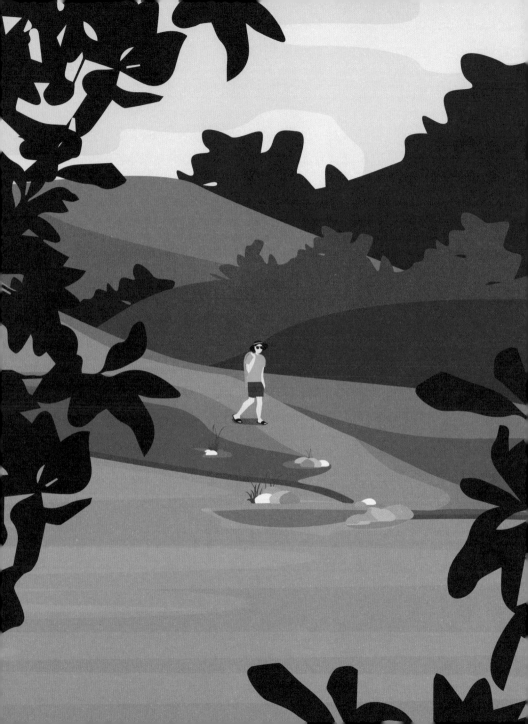

FINDING YOUR PLACE

I was once asked if I had to choose only one place to swim for the rest of my life, would I choose a river, lake, pool, or the sea. It's a tough choice, but I chose the sea. I would really miss river swimming, but the sea has my heart. Every swimmer has a favorite. As well as offering different benefits and experiences, each body of water comes with its own risks, and so the preparation required for each is different. The difficulty with choosing where to swim is often about finding somewhere safe where swimming is allowed. Across the world there are lots of different access and rights-to-roam rules. Sadly, private land often stops play and many countries have some sort of rules around water. Nordic countries like Sweden, Norway, Denmark, and Finland have excellent access and freedom to enjoy the water, while in the UK and parts of America there are lots of access issues. There are various ways to find and discover places to swim, but where do you begin?

Exploring the world

My favorite kind of research is the kind you do yourself. It has taken a while for me to embrace digital maps because I loved having something physically in my hands when out on an adventure, and relying on digital devices out in the wild didn't seem like a good idea. But advances in technology, battery life, and gadgets mean there are plenty of smart ways to navigate. If you have a good sense of direction and can read a map, they are a great way to find swim spots. Bodies of water away from roads and parking tend to be less popular and more tranquil. Even a 30-minute walk can give you a better place to dip than the first sight of water on a public path. Grab a map and look for blue blobs and wiggly river lines. A simple rule is that if you see a sign that says "no swimming," you must respect that.

Swim research
Once you have identified possible walking and swimming routes, do some more research before heading off for a swim.

Bodies of water away from roads and parking tend to be less popular and more tranquil.

→ Use a digital map with a satellite image setting and explore the area virtually before you set out. See if you can identify entry and exit points in the water, and any hazards like grazing cattle or other water users.

→ Use the internet to find out more about an area or body of water. Simply searching for "wild swimming at [location]" can give you information such as any incidents or local issues with swimming in the area.

→ Use social media to search for groups of swimmers in the area. Sometimes you can locate places to swim from photos or group users' posts.

→ Visit the area on foot with a friend and do your own assessment. Pay attention to signage that might indicate dangers, risks, and land ownership.

→ There are guidebooks on swimming that offer written instructions and directions to many different swim spots across the world. Look for books that give you photos, map coordinates, and some background information. Pay attention to when the book was published because swim spot access can change and will be impacted daily due to weather and conditions. I have visited plenty of swim spots from a book that are unsafe—or even without any water!

→ There are some swimming maps online, but they are a bit hit-and-miss. Depending on where they were developed, your country may still look uncharted.

→ There are also a couple of wild swimming apps that replicate books and maps, but at the time of writing are in early development.

Join a group, club, or community

One of the best things about wild swimming is the communities and friendships that have formed around water. I have come across local swimming groups in New York, Chile, Japan, and all over Europe. It appears, no matter where you are in the world, there is usually someone to swim with. If you struggle to find a group, it might be an opportunity for you to start your own. Even inviting a friend to join you can be enough to create a small community. There are wonderful stories worldwide of people who started swimming with just one other, and it soon became a wider group.

A common piece of advice is not to swim alone, mainly so that you can look after each other and call for help if needed. You can swim alone, especially if you know the area and water well, but in a group you can share knowledge and experience, skills, and information. Here are some ways you could find or form a swimming community.

→ Search on social media for groups in your area. A simple "wild swimming [your location]" can throw up options on places like Facebook. Also try searching hashtags on Instagram.

→ If you see people swimming somewhere you'd like to swim, ask if they meet regularly. Swimmers are often quick to offer helpful guidance.

→ Ensure that the group has a similar ability and interest to you. You don't want to join people who are planning to swim long distances if you just want to go for a dip.

→ Be aware of your own ability and limits—don't let group mentality lead you into danger. You should always be responsible for yourself.

→ Use a group to find teachers, coaches, and more experienced swimmers you can learn from. You can even establish goals and share ideas, completing swims together.

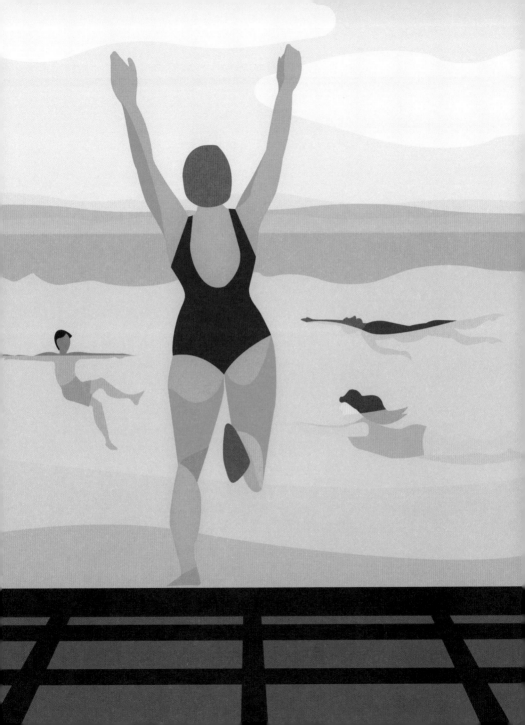

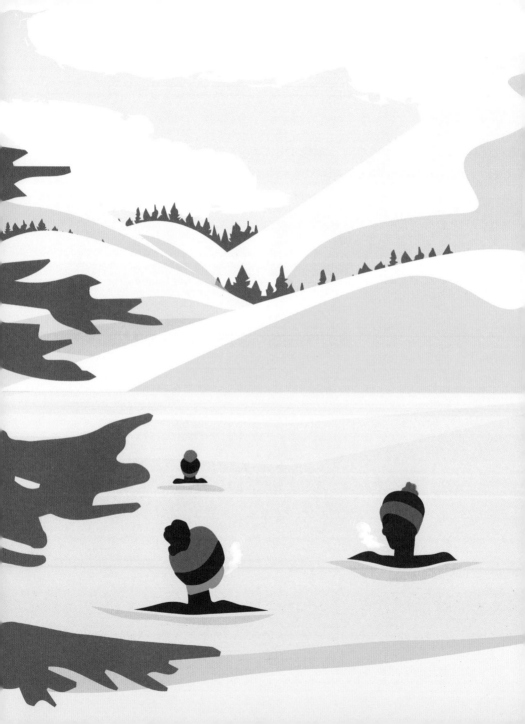

Open-water venues

Public spaces

Supervised open water across the world grew in popularity with triathlons. Open-water venues are generally large lakes located inland. It is common to have facilities like changing areas, toilets, and, if you are lucky, somewhere to get a hot drink and a snack. They are often on private land and managed independently. They provide lifeguards and sometimes offer wetsuit and equipment rental. They are great for beginner outdoor swimmers, training, and for building up confidence. They are also good for learning how to adapt and acclimatize to wild water conditions. The downside is that often they are only open for limited times and days because they usually offer other water sports that clash with swimmers. They also charge to swim.

In very general and broad terms, if you can access water from a public footpath and land, you could argue swimming there is allowed. Laws and rights vary across the world, so it is important to check. Generally, people dip and swim in popular parks and areas the public can access for leisure. But even somewhere small like the UK, the rules vary depending on the country—in Scotland there is a right to roam, while in England there are more restrictions. The US has lots of large national parks, but rangers patrol and can restrict swimming. Much like with our borders across the world, it seems ridiculous that we can't enjoy the land and water, roaming free. But sadly, land is used for many things and some restrictions will be for safety reasons. Pay attention to signage and local laws.

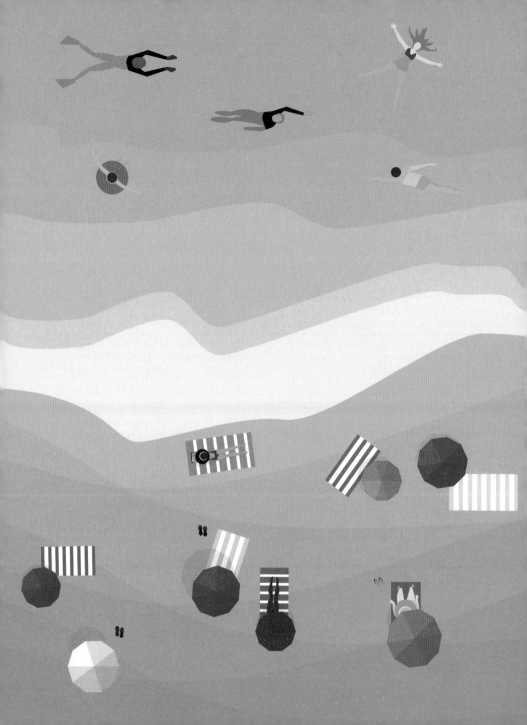

6
BODIES OF WATER

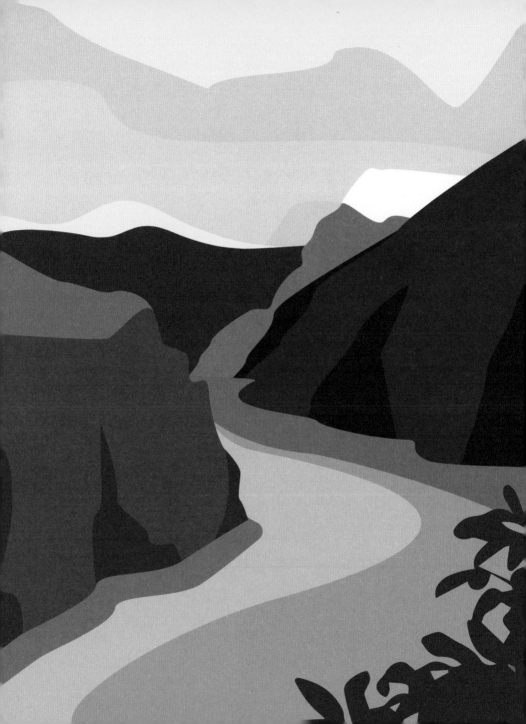

RIVERS, LAKES, PONDS, POOLS, AND SEAS

There is an abundance of types of places you can swim wild, and each one has its advantages, risks, beauty, and hazards. Some bodies of water can change quickly with weather and varying conditions. Some can be strong and invigorating, others more gentle and serene. All of them offer something different and need different preparation. Seasoned wild swimmers tend to have their favorite places to swim and specific spots to enter the water, but as a beginner it is good to head to well-known locations before attempting to discover something more remote or special to you. Each river, lake, pond, pool, or sea has unique elements, and across the world the risks can vary with differences in wildlife, weather, and landscape. Wherever you chose to swim, it is essential that you learn about your local swim spot before dipping in a toe. A freshwater lake in Australia will have very real and different hazards than a lake in England. Likewise with a river in Europe compared to one in South America. But there are some similarities that you can consider and learn about. In this chapter we'll explore what to think about when planning a swim in each of these bodies of water.

The sea

The sea has held people captivated for centuries. It can reset the mind. It can churn us up and spit us out. It perfectly demonstrates the power of nature and the fragility of life. It is human to want to travel across oceans and conquer seas. We love the myths, stories, and mystery of the oceans. They are playgrounds offering long-distance challenge and wild swimming delight. But the sea is home to an abundance of wildlife, and creatures that can snap and sting. It is fickle—one moment a place of peace and the next a swirling danger. When planning a sea swim, think about:

WILDLIFE The sea offers an abundance of wonder and wildlife, some that will harm us to defend themselves. Beaches across the world come with warning signs informing you of risky wildlife native to that area. Pay attention to them. Most things will swim away from you, but jellyfish move with the water, so it is common to encounter them. Enjoy what you can see—dolphins and seals can be fun to swim with, but respect them; it's their home, after all. Learn about common wildlife found in the sea where you want to swim and understand the risks.

TIDES Tidal ranges vary across the world. The UK has one of the biggest tidal ranges in the world, while the Mediterranean and Caribbean seas remain pretty much the same at all times. In very simple terms, the tide is either rising or falling toward a high or low tide. The sea and coastline will be very different at each tide and in between. A high tidal range means that if you head to the coast at low tide, you could be faced with

The sea and coastline will be very different at each tide and in between.

shallow or no water to swim in. At high tide it could be swollen and dangerous. Different rock, stone, and sand at beaches can create different conditions in different tides. There is no simple rule—to swim at only a certain time. The tide times change daily with the moon cycle. The moon causes the tidal movement; and during the month, due to the gravitational pull on the oceans, there will be higher tides (spring tides) and lower tides (neap tides). If you plan to sea swim, find out how the tide affects the area where you want to swim. Search the internet, download apps that chart the tides, or ask local fishermen, lifeguards, or other water users about the water.

WAVES, SWELL, AND CHOP Waves can be fun to jump through or incredibly dangerous. A wave is shaped by the sea floor, wind, tide, and swell. Waves can switch from flat and calm to bouncy and rolling with just a wind change or tidal movement. Often, waves are smaller when the tide is falling

and bigger when the tide is rising. The most challenging thing about waves is that when observing them from the beach, you can never really tell how big they are. It is often only when one swallows you up and tumbles you into a spin that you really understand the force and strength of a wave. It isn't much fun swimming in waves, so if it is rough, unless you want to surf or play, it might be better to skip swimming until calmer conditions arise. Doing some research into the coastline you are visiting will help you figure out whether your chosen spot is better for surfing rather than swimming.

Swell feeds the waves and is the up-and-down motion of the sea, created by weather systems. It can be tough to swim through, but fun too. There are various surfing forecasts that mention swell, wave height, and wind. They are useful for swimmers—high swell usually means rough weather and waves.

Chop, the bouncing water created by the wind and swell, is tough to swim in and adaptations might be needed—like the side you breathe on if swimming front crawl. One overall piece of advice is if the sea looks rough or scary to you, don't swim. Pay attention to your own instincts. They are usually right.

LIFEGUARDED BEACHES The simplest place to start with sea swimming is at lifeguarded beaches, which can be found worldwide. The yellow and red uniform and flags are a global standard, so you can identify a lifeguard station anywhere in the world. Lifeguards not only offer monitoring of the water, but they provide up-to-date information and local knowledge. Even if you don't intend to swim between the flags placed at the beach, a lifeguard station can provide information on tides, weather, wildlife, and other hazards. A lifeguard will know the area well, where rocks are hidden, or if there is a jellyfish bloom present. If you are lucky enough to live in a coastal area, get to know your lifeguard team and share your intended swim routes and plans. If you are a beginner sea swimmer, tell them and they can advise.

WHERE TO ENTER AND EXIT Visit the area at low tide so that you can see what the land is like under the sea. A calm beach could have a deep underwater shelf you can't see, or there may be rocks or dips you are unaware of. The best place to enter the sea is somewhere that starts shallow and allows you to gently walk into deeper water. Some beaches and rocky areas offer steps and rails. Be careful with large waves and swell; this will make entering and exiting the water more challenging and even dangerous. If unsure, always trust that instinct!

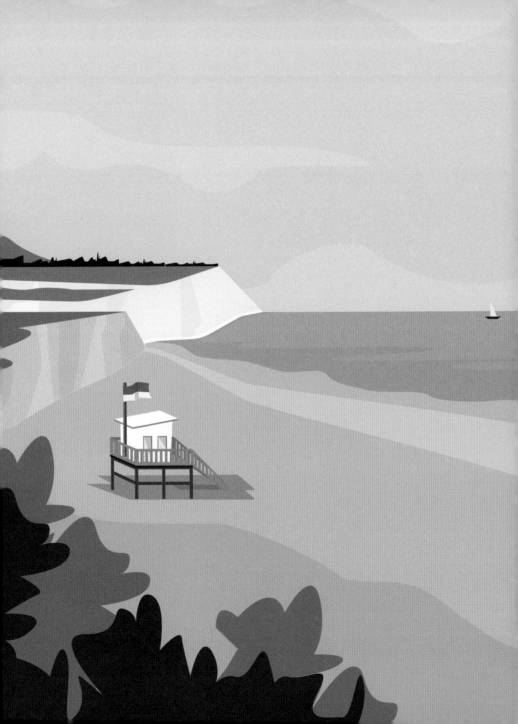

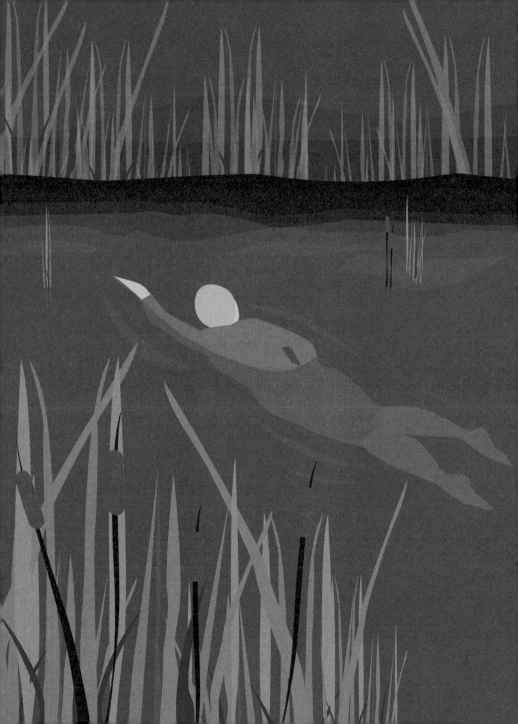

Rivers

Swimming along the river is a wonderful way to explore an area. River journeys are one of my favorite ways to enjoy the water—swimming from one place to another is such a great way to travel.

Rivers can be young and shallow or wide, deep, and meandering. The best way to understand any river is to know where it surfaces at the source and where it is heading. Rivers vary hugely across the world. In the US they can be wide and long, in Australia murky and home to crocodiles, and in Europe blue and cold. They are fantastic fun for paddling, dipping, plunging, or longer swims. When you're planning a river swim, think about:

THE RIVER CATCHMENT This is the area of land surrounding a river where rainwater lands. In mountainous or hilly regions, rivers can fill and rush quickly from heavy rain. Checking the weather upstream as well as where you plan to swim is important—if there is heavy rainfall upstream, it could impact your swim downstream. Equally, in warm seasons, some rivers live underground or dry up completely.

SOURCE OR SEA Water near the source will be colder, either forming from under the ground or ice-melt on mountains. Rivers near the sea will be tidal and brackish – a mix of salt water and fresh water. Tidal parts can be silty and sinking. Do your research!

WHERE TO ENTER AND EXIT Rivers will be moving, even in dry weather. Ensure you know which direction the water is traveling—with currents, eddies, rocks, and swirls, it isn't always clear. If you intend to get out where you get in, swim upstream, but ensure you have a plan to exit farther downstream from your planned exit point regardless—often the strength of the river can be surprising and hard to swim against. It is best to enter in a place where you can do so gradually. Wading into the river will enable you to feel the strength of the current around your ankles before

Ensure you know which direction the water is traveling—with currents, eddies, rocks, and swirls, it isn't always clear.

swimming out of your depth. Riverbanks can be steep and sometimes dense with plant life, so it isn't always as easy to exit a river as it is to enter.

UNDERWATER HAZARDS Boulders, rocks, branches, and litter can obstruct or batter you in the water. Don't jump or dive into a river unless you have tested the depth first.

THE SPEED OF THE WATER Water travels faster when it is shallow or narrow in young rivers. On straight sections of a wide river the middle will have the fastest flow; on bends the outer edges will be where the current is at its strongest.

WEIRS AND WATERFALLS There are natural formations on rivers, but also man-made ones. Weirs and waterfalls can be tempting and fun places to swim, offering jacuzzi bubbles and river pools beneath. But be careful of white water—water with air bubbles in it— because we are less buoyant in it and

therefore more likely to sink. Swim out to the side from white water, rather than directly up to the surface.

WEATHER AND POLLUTION Rivers are impacted by pollution and debris after heavy rainfall. Everything gets washed into our rivers. Don't swim in swollen or flooded rivers, or after spells of persistent or heavy rainfall. In addition to poor water quality, you are more likely to encounter debris that could interfere with your swimming.

WILDLIFE In some parts of the world there are river creatures that can harm humans. Plants too can sting and cause rashes. Just make sure you understand the risks before plunging in.

Lakes and ponds

Lakes, ponds, tarns, reservoirs, fjords, and lochs all have one defining quality: they are bodies of water that have little movement or current. They can be man-made or formed from melting ice, moving rock, or volcanoes. With varying depths, fed by streams, rivers, or ground springs, they are fantastic places to swim. Large lakes are popular for swimming across or around, paddling in, or other leisure activities. They can be owned or wild in national parks. High mountain lakes can be cold and deep, lower-land lakes murky or boggy. Large lakes can act like the ocean, affected by wind and chop. While some are shallow and warm quickly in summer, others are deep with drop-offs and very cold water. When planning a lake swim think about:

WEATHER AND CONDITIONS Wind and rain will make lake swimming more challenging because the water will be choppier. Hot weather can create soupy, weedy conditions in shallow lakes, and in cold weather they can freeze over.

WHERE TO ENTER AND EXIT As with all outdoor swimming, ensure you know where you will enter and exit before getting in. The best entry spot in a lake is from a beach area, where the water starts shallow and drops off. This way you can enter carefully and at your own pace. Some lakes with surrounding rocks might have natural rock steps in and out of the water. Don't use sloping shingle edges; these can be a slip hazard on entry and very difficult to climb up after your swim.

YOUR ABILITY As with any body of water, swim within your ability. Don't go out of your depth if you can't swim well. Don't jump or dive in unless you have tested the depth.

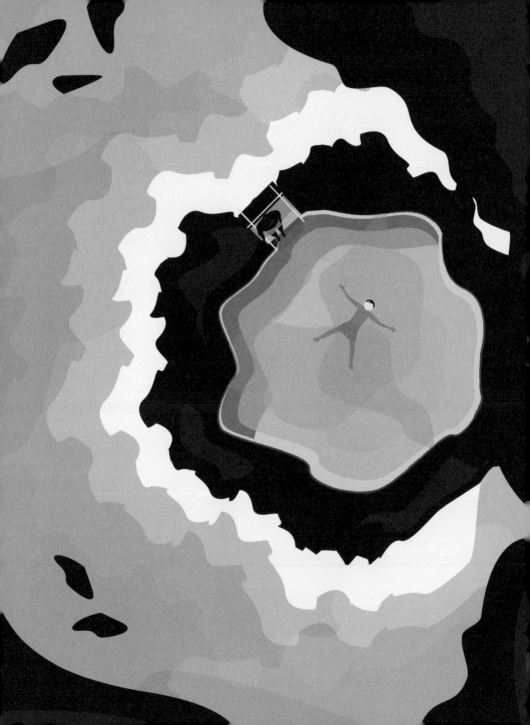

Pools

Outdoor pools, lidos, and tidal pools are a great place for beginner wild swimmers. They are cold and open to the elements, but usually offer entry and exit ladders and facilities. Many are also lifeguarded. While it may seem odd to mention pools in a book about wild swimming, there are some wonderful wild pools in the world. In the Azores, the Portuguese archipelago in the middle of the Atlantic, there are naturally formed tidal pools that make excellent swimming spots. They are filled with wildlife and the cold Atlantic Ocean but contained and protected from the swell.

There are also numerous beautiful river pools all over the world that form at the bottom of waterfalls, above weirs, and as the land changes downhill in young rivers around boulders. They can be a fun, safe place to play and dip. You may see rope hanging from trees where people have swung and plunged in. These little pools are shaped by the river and weather, and as such they can change between visits, so always check the depth before jumping in.

Man-made outdoor pools are also a great way to acclimatize to cooler water and get used to swimming in wind, rain, and even snow!

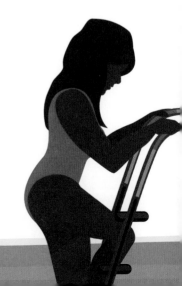

7

RISKS!
IS IT
SAFE?

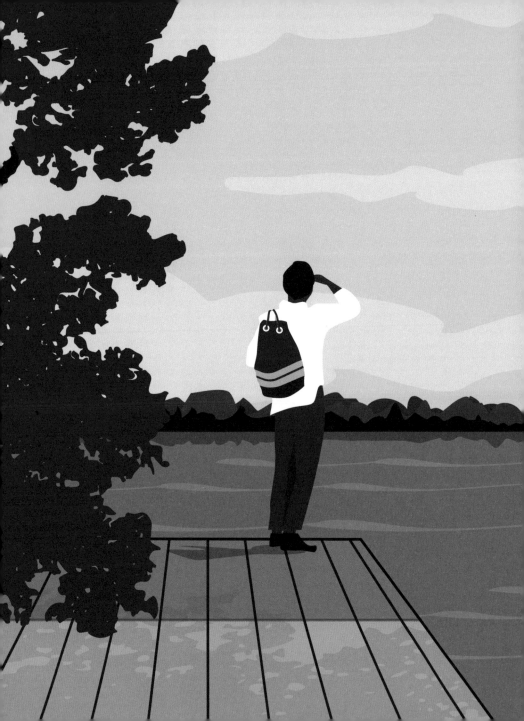

ASSESSING THE RISKS

Like any outdoor activity, wild swimming comes with an element of risk—the unpredictably of water is part of what makes it so appealing and magical, but it is important to learn how to mitigate the risks. Once you know you can swim, float, and tread water (see pages 28–35), the best way to keep yourself safe is by learning how to make a personal risk assessment every time you swim, particularly if it's a new place or you're swimming there under different circumstances and in varying weather conditions. As we covered in the preceding two chapters, where you are swimming will determine your planning and preparation—different bodies of water pose a different set of risks. Here we'll take a look at various hazards associated with wild swimming and the precautions you can take to keep yourself safe in the water.

The drowning chain

The foundation of lifeguard training is the drowning chain. It shows four key elements that can lead to drowning. If you remove one or more of the links, it is less likely that someone will drown.

→ Lack of education
→ Lack of safety advice and protection
→ Lack of safety supervision
→ Inability to cope once in difficulty

When assessing risk in wild swimming, a lack of education is common with accidents and incidents. Not knowing about, ignoring, or misjudging danger is easily done when being spontaneous or enjoying the water with friends. It is important to remember that you are responsible for your own ability and actions.

Trust your instincts

You know that icky, can't-put-your-finger-on-it feeling you sometimes get? When the pit of your stomach says something isn't right? Trust that! Our senses can also aid our instincts. I often tell swimmers that if something doesn't look, sound, smell, feel, or even taste right around water, it probably isn't. In particular, pay attention if you decide to jump, dive, or swim somewhere unfamiliar, or out of your depth.

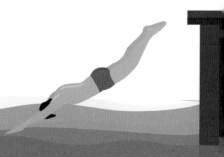

Common risks

Each body of water and location will come with different risks to plan for and mitigate (see page 99). If heading to the coast, you need to consider tides; if you are going to swim in a river, you need to think about flow rate and cleanliness. In different parts of the world there are various animals and plant life that we need to be aware of. The variations are endless, but following are some of the common risks you can consider on location, wherever you choose to swim.

Water quality
It is rare to find natural water free of pathogens. Naturally occurring bacteria, plant, and animal life will impact water quality as well as pollution from road and agricultural runoff. While it might not be good enough to drink, water can still be clean enough to bathe in. There are some simple, natural clues to look for. Water that is clean enough to swim in shouldn't smell bad. If you can see an abundance of wildlife, hear birds, and see fish, these are all good indicators of healthy water. Insects like dragonflies, water boatmen, and damselflies don't like dirty water, so they are great to see on a river. Watch out for rainbow fuel swirls and brown foam, which are indicators of pollution.

Weather and conditions
There is more detail in Chapter 9, but in simple terms weather can change a swimming experience. Too cold, too hot, wet, windy, or icy—they all come with risks.

Entry and exit points
Ensuring there are safe entry and exit points is essential. Sometimes it is easier to get in than to get out.

Water and air temperature
Temperatures can put you at risk for hyperthermia (see page 110) or hypothermia (see pages 106–107). It will impact what you choose to swim in and the equipment you take with you. It will also affect your swimming ability and time you should spend in the water. See the next chapter for more details.

Tides, currents, flow

Which way is the river flowing? Is it fast flowing? Are there hidden currents or any unusual movements? If the tide is coming in, you could get cut off, or belongings left on a beach might be washed away.

Depth of water

How deep is the water? Can you put your feet down? How long until you're out of your depth? Is it deep enough to jump in?

Conditions underfoot

What is the ground like where you are swimming? Is it sandy, gravelly, muddy, or weedy? Keep in mind that spiky sea urchins, shells, and rockfish like shallow water around rocks in the sea.

Hazards in the water

Look out for hazards you can see, like buoys or boats, and be careful of unseen underwater hazards like rocks, weeds, or litter.

Plant and animal life

Depending on where you plan to swim, there will be different wildlife to consider. For example, jellyfish in the sea and stinging nettles on a riverbank are two mild risks, but different countries have various natural hazards, some more serious than others. Generally, most things in the water will swim away from you, but there are plenty of examples where swimming with wildlife is risky. Even a seal can be dangerous—when they are not hunting animals, they are playful and act like puppies in the water, but a bite from a seal can be nasty.

Depending on where you plan to swim, there will be different wildlife to consider.

Pollution

Sadly, pollution is a common problem across the world. This can be found in many forms—floating litter like plastics and fishing nets, fuel leaks from motorboats, sewage leaked from land pipes, and runoff from industry or agriculture. Human action can pose a big risk for wild swimmers. There are organizations across the world campaigning for better water quality and fighting against ocean pollution. Some of these organizations also produce useful maps that inform swimmers of sewage issues in local coastal areas. Polluted water can make you ill if consumed or if it gets into your system through a cut or scrape on the skin.

Other water users

People fishing, boats, personal watercraft, surfers, paddleboarders, and even other swimmers can all be hazards for you to consider when entering wild water. Fast-moving craft might not be able to see you in the water.

Personal health and ability

How are you feeling today? Have you slept well? Have you eaten and drunk fluids? Seems obvious, but if you don't feel great, your swim won't be great. Often, if you are tired you can feel the cold more. If you are cold or not well before you get into the water, you could make things worse.

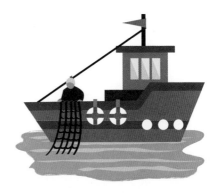

Mitigating risks

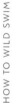

What does this mean? Well, this is where you take a few moments at your chosen location and look for hazards, evaluate the risks, and decide on precautions. As well as planning what to take with you when off for a wild dip, you should pay attention to changing conditions and circumstances. There have been several times I have planned a swim and the weather forecast was wrong, or the entry and exit points had changed since I last swam at the location. The following table covers the common hazards and outlines how you can think about them in terms of risk and how to mitigate it.

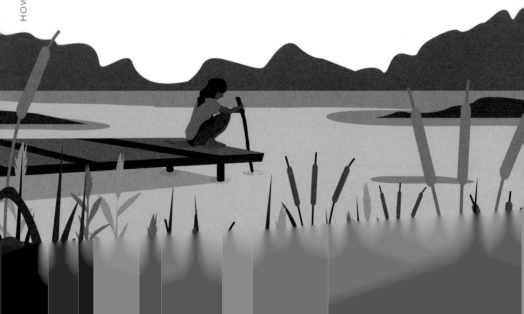

HAZARD	RISK	PRECAUTION
Water quality	Poor water quality can lead to illness.	Don't swim after heavy rainfall. Cover cuts and scrapes. Try not to consume any water.
Weather and conditions	Wind, rain, ice, and heat can all create challenging swimming conditions.	Check the forecast ahead of swimming and ensure those that plan to swim have the capability to do so in challenging conditions.
Entry and exit points	Might be slippery or too steep to enter and exit safely.	Wear appropriate footwear and plan before entering the water
Water and air temperature	Cold weather and water can lead to hypothermia. Hot weather can lead to hyperthermia.	Prepare warm clothes for after swimming or ensure your swimwear has UV protection, stay hydrated, and limit swim time.
Tides, currents, flow	Unknown water direction can lead to panic or difficulty in the water.	Check high and low tide times before entering the sea or tidal rivers.
Depth of water	Shallow water can lead to injury when jumping in.	Test the depth before jumping into water.
Conditions underfoot	Cuts, scrapes, or something stuck into skin on foot.	Wear appropriate footwear to protect soft skin on feet.
Hazards in the water	Swimming into or being struck by an obstruction in the water.	Visually assess water before entering. Use goggles when in the water.
Plant and animal life	Being stung, bitten, or developing a rash.	Check for common wildlife and plant life at the location where you plan to swim.
Pollution	Becoming ill or reacting to polluted water.	Check local authority maps and information at location. Do a visual/sensory check before entering water.
Other water users	Not being seen by other water users, colliding with them.	Inform other users of your swimming plans and route. Wear a bright hat and use a bright tow float so that you can be seen.
Personal health and ability	Not being able to swim as far or as well. Making an existing condition worse.	Ensure you feel fit and well before entering the water.

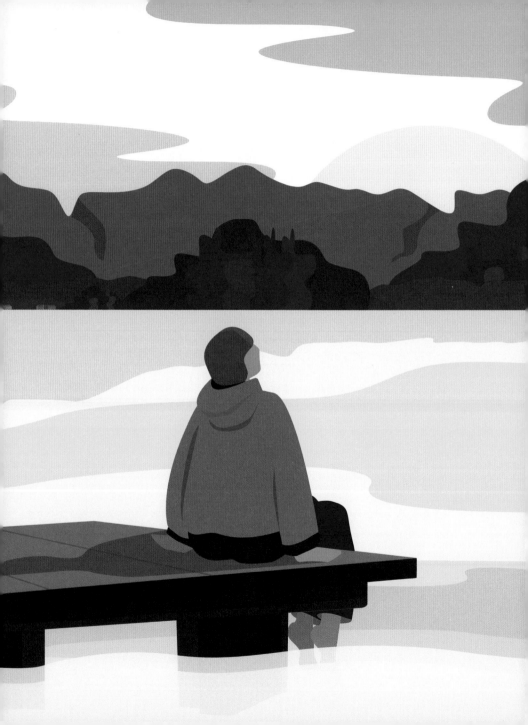

8

HOT AND COLD CONDITIONS

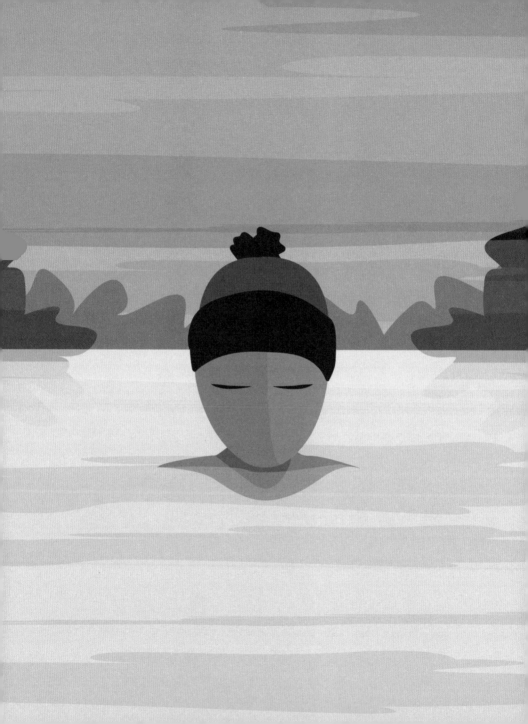

SWIMMING ALL YEAR ROUND

Outdoor swimming is popular during seasons when the air is warm and a cool dip in wild water can relieve hot, sticky skin. For years I only swam outdoors between May and October, returning to pools in winter months. After I trained for a long-distance swim in cooler water, I realized how much I was missing by limiting my wild swims to half the year. Learning how to swim in different conditions and adapting to cold water extended my swimming to year-round enjoyment.

Cold-water swimming and immersion has recently seen a rise in popularity across the world. As well as some small studies into the benefits, there is lots of anecdotal evidence of how swimming outdoors can aid overall well-being. People who swim in wintery conditions across the world report both physical and mental benefits. Wild swimmers claim to be more resilient, productive, and positive if they regularly swim outdoors. Swimming outside at any time can improve mood, strengthen your immune system, and relieve stress.

I encourage anyone who wants to try cold-water swimming to start when the weather is warm and conditions are calmer. If you live in a country that cools as the seasons change, start swimming in warmer seasons and then continue to swim as the water and weather cool. It can be uncomfortable when you first dip into water below 50˚F (10˚C), but on the other side of that discomfort is the zing! Let's look at swimming in cold and hot conditions.

Cold-water swimming

Technically, all water below body temperature can feel cold. All wild water will be significantly cooler than your core body temperature, so understanding how your body responds to this is essential when swimming outdoors. This is before considering other conditions like air temperature and weather. Anything below 59°F (15°C) is considered cold water, but most of us will feel anything under 68°F (20°C) as cold. We are all individuals with different biological makeups, so there aren't blanket rules or standard responses to the cold—it will be different for everyone. If you carry more body fat, you will feel warmer than some, but if you haven't eaten, feel cold before entering the water, or are very tired, you might feel colder than your fellow swimmers. There are some common reactions we all have when entering cool water. If we regularly swim outdoors, we can get better at managing them, but our bodies will still be responding. The following pages cover things to watch out for.

Cold-water shock

Cold-water shock is an instant reaction when entering cold water. A swimmer will often gasp, taking a large breath and finding it hard to exhale or control breathing. It can cause panic if not expected. If you jump into cold water, this gasp reaction can happen under the water, which puts you at a higher risk of drowning. To overcome this shock, it is best to enter the water slowly but consistently. Enter within your depth and pay attention to your breathing. Get your shoulders under the water while you're still in your depth so you can control your breathing before lifting off into a swim. It is important to just focus on regular, calm breathing—no need for deep breaths or anything fancy. This will gently calm your body and send the message to your brain that this immersion is intentional. Entering cold water will feel uncomfortable to begin with. The discomfort will pass. Cold-water shock can occur for anyone at any time; this doesn't just happen to winter swimmers.

Swim failure

As you enter cool water and get your breathing under control, remember that your body will still be continuing to cool. Swimming, moving your body, and exerting yourself in the water will generate some body heat, but your body will still be losing heat to the water. The colder the water, the quicker the heat loss. Initially when swimming in cool water, it is our skin that loses heat, which then triggers the cold water shock response. But as we swim, our muscles can start to cool, too. This is more common in very cold water, but can happen to anyone at any time. As our nerves and muscles cool, we can feel weaker, and our swimming can slow or fail. It is common for this to occur in our arms first, so noticing loss of efficiency in your arms is a good indicator that it is time to get out. The risk of swim failure depends on many variables, but it is worth knowing the signs so you can recognize when you need to exit the water as quickly as possible to go and warm up.

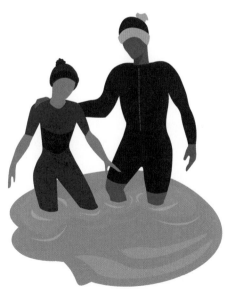

Hypothermia

In simple terms, hypothermia is when your core body temperature drops below 95°F (35°C). Our bodies in normal, resting conditions keep a regular core temperature of around 99°F (37°C). When your body loses heat quicker than it can generate it, a heat deficit develops and core body temperature falls. Swimming in cold water increases the speed of heat loss, and prolonged periods in the water can lead to overall body temperature drop. Water surrounding the body pulls heat out through conduction. How our bodies respond to the cold and protect us from hypothermia can be influenced by air temperature, dehydration, lack of nutrition, body fat, and acclimatization. Even after we leave the water, our body temperature can continue to drop, so the risk of hypothermia continues until we are dressed and warming up again.

You can reduce the risk of hypothermia by planning your swim effectively and also by learning about your own body

Signs and symptoms

— Pale skin, blue lips

— Shivering and then muscle stiffness

— Slowing body functions—struggling with speech and thought

— Slurred speech

— Confusion or disorientation

— Slow to respond to instructions or help

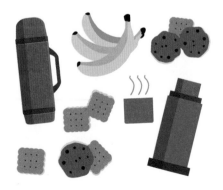

through short periods of exposure to cold water. It is different for everyone, but I know I feel colder if I have an empty stomach or haven't slept well the night before. Also, if the sun is out, I can withstand colder water for longer than if it is cloudy or windy. I only know this through experiencing it myself, by gently extending my time in the water and learning my body's response.

If you or anyone you swim with recognizes the signs of hypothermia—we often see it in others before we see it in ourselves—it is important to act quickly. Get the swimmer out of the water to a sheltered area, or indoors. Dry and dress them and cover them with warm blankets. Foil blankets are only useful as a last outer layer over warmer fabrics in these circumstances. Get the swimmer inside—a car is great if you're not near any buildings. Turn the heaters on and give the swimmer a warm drink, with something sweet like cookies or chocolate.

Reduce the risks

— Ensure you have a hot drink in a flask ready for after your swim.

— Pack plenty of dry, warm clothes—multiple layers including a good thermal base layer.

— Have a warm hat to put on as soon as you get out.

— Before swimming, prepare your clothes for after the swim. Put them in the order you will need them and ensure they are all at hand.

— A decent warm coat will be a good investment. Padded and longer coats that are made with wind- and waterproof materials are ideal.

— A changing robe (see page 63) can be useful for protecting you from the elements as you get dressed in cool conditions.

Afterdrop

When you first enter cold water, it is your extremities and the surface of your skin that cool first and quickest, but over time the cooling spreads to your core. Even after you have left the water, the cold will continue to spread and cool your body. Studies have shown that this drop in core temperature can continue for twenty to thirty minutes after a swim. Swimmers call this afterdrop. So, while you could have had a great swim, exited the water safely, and be getting dressed, you could still encounter afterdrop. It is essential that you are dry, dressed, and warming to mitigate the effects of afterdrop. Despite leaving the water feeling elated and wonderful, don't waste time in this state. I often see swimmers chatting and standing around in just their swimsuits dripping wet, unaware their bodies are still cooling fast. It is harder to dress when you are shivering and shaking, so dry and dress quickly.

Cramping

Cramping is when muscles go into spasm. It is most common in lower limbs when you are tired, or your muscles get cold—I really suffer in my calf muscles. When it happens in open water it can cause panic and make you thrash about. It can be painful and hard to stretch out a cramp when you're in the water. Rolling onto your back and trying to stretch the muscle can help; using a tow float to rest on can be useful too. Using your arms to swim into shallow water so you can stand and stretch is also good. If you are with another swimmer, they can help you get to within your depth. Keeping well hydrated and regularly engaging in a complementary exercise like yoga out of the water can also be useful.

Cuts and bruises

When our skin is numb and cold, our sensitivity to pain is reduced. If you choose to swim in icy conditions, be aware that ice can cut or puncture skin, often without us noticing. Equally, swimming into underwater hazards can cause bruising that we may not notice until later once we have warmed up. When swimming in cold water, take extra care and protect your feet. You might not feel the discomfort of jabbing stones when you can't feel your feet!

Swimmer's and surfer's ear

There are two risks with ears and cold-water exposure. First is a bacterial risk, where cool water enters the ear and can remain, creating an infection. This can be resolved with eardrops from a pharmacist or doctor. Infections are rare, though and it is normal to get water in your ears, which can remain inside even after getting out of the water. It can feel and sound like a feather inside your ear canal. Simply laying down on the ear that is affected and waiting for it to trickle out will solve it. The other risk is commonly known as surfer's ear. This condition is caused by repeated exposure to cold water and wind. It causes bony growth to develop in the ear, which can lead to hearing loss and infections. Both these risks can be mitigated with the use of earplugs and by wearing a swim cap.

Even after you have left the water, the cold will continue to cool your body.

Swimming in the heat

As the climate changes across the world, more of us are dealing with hotter weather than we are used to. While a cool swim sounds ideal in a heatwave, there are risks when swimming in hot weather. Being outside in very little clothing, like most swimwear, we are at higher risk of sun exposure and hyperthermia. Swimming regularly outdoors can lead to an increased risk of skin cancer, so wear waterproof sunscreen and swimwear that offers UV protection.

Hyperthermia

Commonly known as heatstroke, hyperthermia is when the body core temperature exceeds 104°F (40°C). Swimming for long periods of time in hot climates or for long distances in warm water can put you at higher risk. Also, if you wear a wetsuit you are more likely to overheat in warmer weather and water. If you notice yourself or someone else displaying the symptoms of hyperthermia, move them to a cool, shaded area and give them fluids.

Signs and symptoms

— Hot, red, and dry skin

— Headache

— Dizziness, fainting, and light-headedness

— Confusion and/or slow to respond

— Nausea and/or vomiting

Reduce the risks

— Avoid swimming during the hottest part of the day

— Have shorter dips rather than long swims

— Ensure you are well hydrated; you don't notice sweat in the water

— Use tinted goggles

— Swim without a wetsuit

— Wear sunscreen and UV swimwear

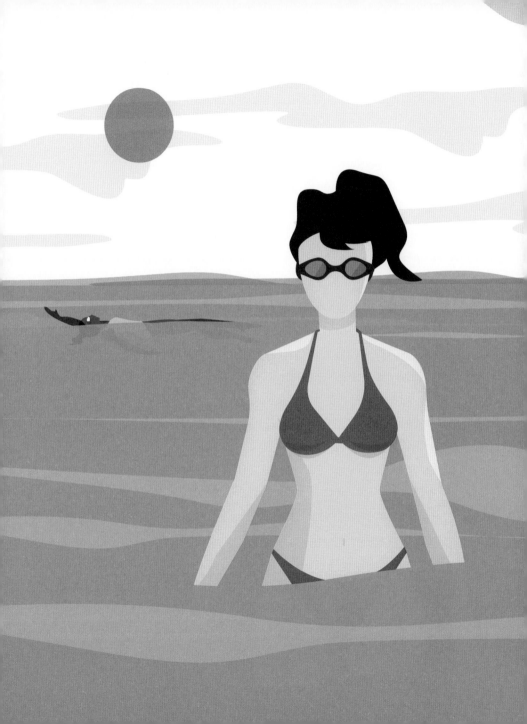

Weeds and algae

Warm, sunny weather increases the plant life in water, particularly in shallow areas of the sea, rivers, and shallow lakes. Open-water venues combat weeds and algae with natural dyes to diffuse sunlight and thus prevent growth, and some use weed cutters. But wild swimming locations are—well—wild. Shallow rivers will see a bloom of weeds in warm weather—not only are they growing under sunny conditions, but water levels will drop when there is less rainfall. Weeds are largely just unpleasant to swim through, but can also cause panic, which can lead to legs and arms getting tangled. If you encounter weeds, try to float through them, remaining calm so that you can extract yourself.

If you encounter weeds, try to float through them, remaining calm so that you can extract yourself.

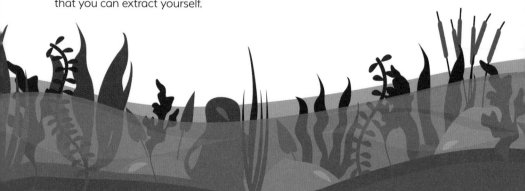

Warm water will also see other growth like algae. Some algae, such as cyanobacteria, named blue-green algae because of its color, can grow toxic blooms. It grows inland in water that has little flow or current, like lakes and ponds. Blue-green algae is part of the natural ecosystem, but when it reproduces rapidly into blooms it can cover surface area quickly and releases toxins. It impacts the color and clarity of the water and can be fatal to dogs, as well as cause skin rashes for some swimmers. You can spot the blue-green color like paint in the water, and it sometimes creates surface scum. If you see signs of this algae, find somewhere else to swim.

Swimmer's itch

Another natural phenomenon in warmer water is something called swimmer's itch. There is no tactful way to describe this—it is a skin reaction to a tiny parasitic worm that tries to burrow into your skin. Its intended targets are ducks and other water birds. It can't live in humans or enter your bloodstream, but it can leave a small red bump like an insect bite. It is more common in warmer seasons, but can occur in winter. Swimming in warm or weedy water can increase the chance of encountering swimmer's itch. As with other insect bites, some people are more affected than others. Swimming in deeper water, wearing a wetsuit, and showering after swimming can help. If you encounter the itch, antihistamine creams and tablets can help—don't scratch!

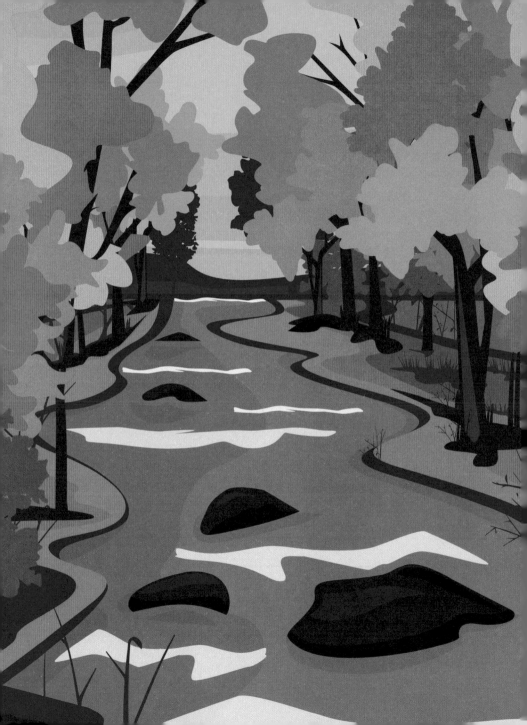

9

THE
SEASONS
AND
WEATHER

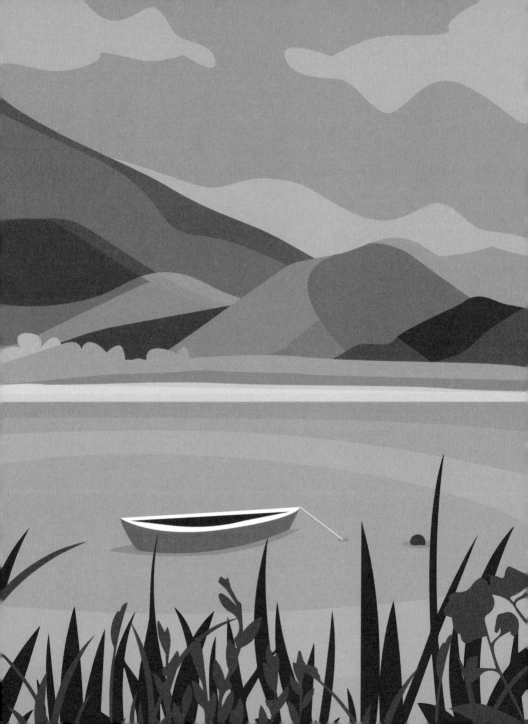

SEASONAL AND CELESTIAL SWIMS

I love swimming in spring, but each season has its charms, wildlife, flowers, fauna, and risks. Wild swimming year-round, all through the seasons, under full moons, and during solar events creates connection to the natural world. You notice the hopeful buds in deep winter and can sense the cooler season coming at the end of summer. You become attuned to natural clues and can identify when something isn't right or is unseasonable. It is perhaps why wild swimmers work hard to protect locations from litter, why they comb beaches for treasures and trash, or prune, protect, and sow seeds on riverbanks. While there are some parts of the world that don't experience four distinct seasons like I do in the UK, wherever you are in the world, I hope you embrace swimming in the changing seasons, appreciating the beautiful natural world around you.

Spring

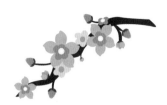

Wild water in spring is cold after the winter, yet to warm up. So, when the days start to get warmer and brighter, if you wake early you can catch a mist hovering above the water. Plants unfurl, the air smells sweet, spring flowers and tree blossoms carpet the ground. Water clarity is good, warmer air temperature allows for slightly longer swims, and you can leave a few extra layers at home. Warmer days than expected can ignite spontaneous swims, and increased daylight hours allow time for more play.

Rain

Swimming in the rain is immersive and sensory. Rain on the surface of the water you are swimming in creates patterns and ripples that are mesmerizing. Water above, below, and around, it is a complete immersion in nature. However, it comes with some risks and considerations. If the forecast predicts rain, ensure you have a decent duffel bag or somewhere to put your dry gear for after your swim. Not being able to dry and dress can make you cold and at risk for hypothermia (see pages 106–107). Prolonged rain can affect water quality, increase runoff, and create debris in the water. In some areas, rain can quickly change the flow and depth of a river.

Fog

Foggy and misty conditions are more common between changing seasons like winter into spring and fall into winter. In simple terms, it is low-lying cloud. A high density of water droplets is created by cooler and warmer air mixing. It can be beautiful, but as on dry land, it decreases visibility, so other water users can't see you as well and it is easy to become disoriented. In large areas of open water like seas, lakes, and some rivers, you might not be able to see the water's edge, the direction you want to swim in, or the place that you're trying to reach. Consider additional visibility measures like waterproof lights and tow floats, but don't swim in thick fog.

Summer

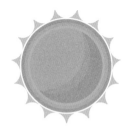

This is the most popular season for wild swimming. Fair-weather swimmers flock to their nearest swimming spots to cool off and enjoy the sunshine. If you swim all year round it can be annoying to find your swimming spot crowded or, even worse, ruined by anti-social behavior. Water that is easy to get to by car or public transportation will be busier, so take time to walk to spots out of popular reach. Summer can be a great time to start your wild swimming, when the water is warmer and more inviting and there are more options for safe swimming—like lifeguarded beaches. Light mornings and evenings allow extended time to enjoy the water.

Sun

Hot weather can increase cold water shock (see page 104), as the water will be cooler than the air temperature. Also, sunshine can cause sunburn and heatstroke (see page 110). Dry conditions can also mean less water—some lakes and rivers dry up in summer.

Electrical storms

Warm weather brings a higher risk of thunder and lightning. Never swim in an electrical storm—lightning often strikes the tallest local object, so when you are in open water, that is likely to be you! Water also conducts electricity, so if you are not hit directly, you could still be harmed by a nearby strike. If you hear thunder or see lightning, exit the water. Don't enter again until thirty minutes have passed since the last rumble of thunder or lightning flash.

Fall

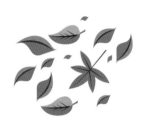

As in spring, fall can bring misty conditions. This time the water has been warmed by the summer sun, and cooler air temperatures create the magical mist across the water. Fall is favored by many wild swimmers because the water remains warm, but cooler conditions discourage fair-weather swimmers. It means longer swims can continue, but with fewer water users to encounter. Falling leaves and autumnal colur adds a new dimension to wild water. Leaves swirling between fingers and around you as you swim is special. Occasional cool days with frost and turbulent weather is a stark reminder that winter is on its way.

Wind

Water becomes livelier in windy conditions. In open water such as the sea and large lakes, it will create chop, waves, and swell (see pages 81–82). This can make swimming more interesting, but also exhausting and sometimes dangerous. Wind can cool you down more quickly, so pay special attention to wind chill in cooler months. Also, wind can blow down branches and sweep things into the water, so watch out for debris.

Cold

After a summer of warm swims, it might take some time to adjust to the cooler air and water temperatures fall brings. Shorten your swims and start planning for colder water, packing extra layers to be used if needed. A few days of very cold weather can cool down water temperature quickly, so even if you swam a couple of days ago, a significant change of conditions could have occurred since.

Winter

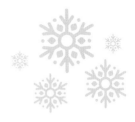

Swimming in winter is for a select few. In some countries, swimming is reduced to dips in ice holes, but wherever you are, winter swims will be shorter. Officially, ice swimming can be done in any water at 41˚F (5˚C) or under. With a warming climate, some parts of the world are experiencing warmer winters, so cold water is becoming harder to find for ice swimmers. Swimming in winter is uncomfortable and wonderful in equal measures. Dedicating yourself to winter swimming forces you to get out in nature when many other people are tucked up indoors. It creates social groups that connect people during the loneliest months and helps tackle seasonal depression and mental health issues.

Snow and ice

Cold air and water temperatures put you at risk of cold water shock, swim failure, hypothermia, afterdrop, cramp, numbness, and ear infections (see pages 104–109). Snow and ice also create difficult transportation conditions, so putting yourself at risk when emergency services might not reach you is something to think about avoiding. Short swims, with planning, can be joyful while it is snowing. Just ensure you have plenty of warm, dry clothes for afterwards and something hot to drink.

Dark

Winter brings shorter days and longer spells of darkness. Some places never see daylight in winter, and so swimming in the dark might be the only option available. Water is different at night. Not being able to see what is in the water or around you can be alluring and exciting. Ensure you are visible, though—waterproof swim lights can be attached to goggles or tow floats. Leave a light where you plan to enter and exit the water and swim somewhere familiar to reduce the risk of trips and falls.

Moons

Equinox and solstice

Swimming around the cycles of the moon can be a lovely ritual and a great routine to get into. Full and new moons bring high spring tides at the coast, and the full moon can provide a brightly lit, glittering path across dark water under clear skies. There are many cultures that traditionally celebrate and mark full moons—wild swimmers have embraced the ritual, and some even swim naked under them. Mark the full moons in your calendar and figure out where the moon will rise at your swim spot, then join in swim-howling at the moon.

Following the seasonal and natural cycles becomes easier when swimming outdoors. The Wheel of the Year, celebrated and followed by pagans, uses nature to connect to the divine. Equinoxes mark the beginning of each quarter, closely linked to the seasons, and solstices mark midsummer and midwinter. The cycle can be used to align your life with the rhythms of nature, which could be done with wild swimming. Sunrise and sunset swims are popular with wild swimmers around equinox and solstice.

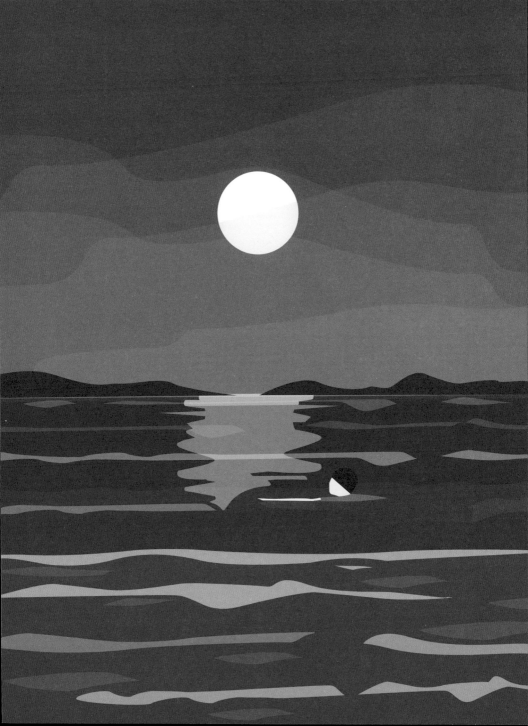

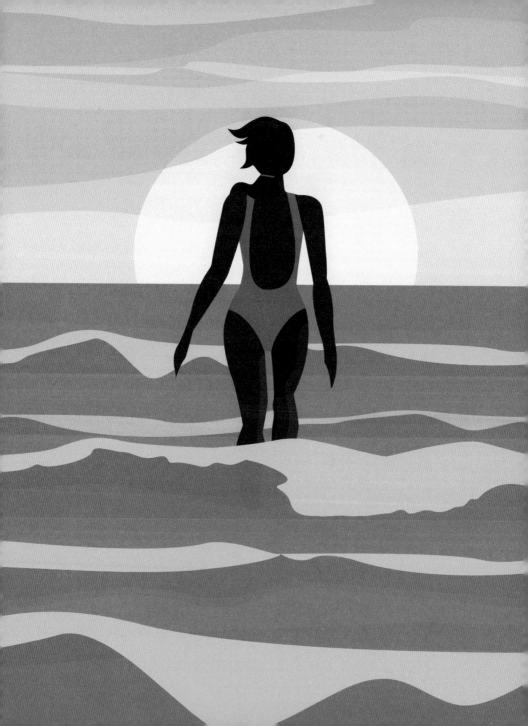

10
PREPARING
TO
SWIM

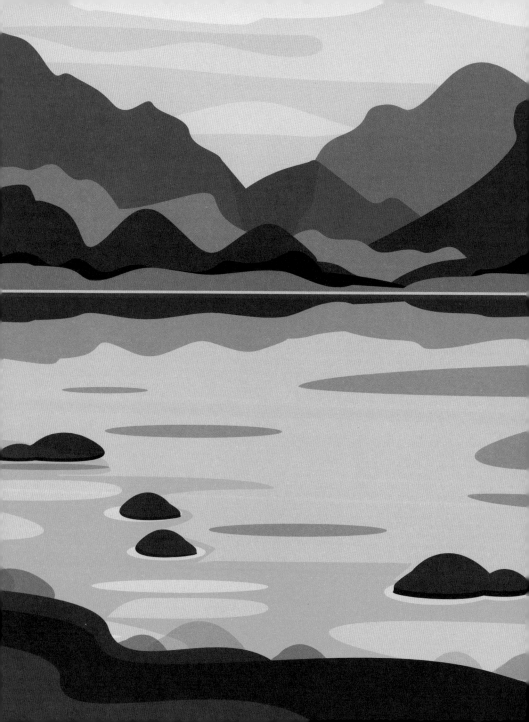

FORMING THE FOUNDATIONS

At the beginning of your wild swimming journey there are so many questions. What should I wear? Is it safe? Where should I swim? Who should I go with? If you haven't undertaken proper preparation and your head is still swirling with these questions by the time you are at the water's edge, you might be filled with fear. While I may sound like a bore to constantly prompt new wild swimmers to plan, prepare, and assess, the more you swim wild, the more these things become habit and instinct, so you can then swim more spontaneously. You will understand your ability and body in water, what it feels like to swim in different conditions, and how you deal with the unpredictability of water, as well as factors you can mitigate. All the questions you try to answer in the beginning will form the foundations that will enable you to swim wild.

Planning your swim

When you arrive at your chosen swim location, don't forget to do a quick visual risk assessment (see pages 98–99). Taking a moment to assess the area before swimming can make it more enjoyable as well as safer. Refer back to all the previous chapters in this book and use the following prompts to plan a swim:

Where am I going?
What's your knowledge of the area? How will you get there? Is any further research required?

Who am I going with?
Think about swimming ability and confidence. Can everyone stay within their safe limits?

What sort of swim am I doing?
Are you thinking of a dip or a float, long-distance, or a journey from one place to another?

What are the conditions?
Consider the weather forecast, tides, water conditions, and temperature.

What will I need?
Swimsuit or wetsuit, towel, clothes, footwear, map, flask, sunscreen? See pages 39–65 to remind yourself of the equipment you might need.

What are the risks?
What are the risks in your chosen location? Consider how you can mitigate them and plan for success (see pages 93–99).

Taking a moment to assess the area before swimming can make it more enjoyable as well as safer.

Respecting the environment

Many of the best swimming locations are wild and beautiful, which is why you want to swim there. Try to respect the environment, wildlife, and plant life while you are visiting. Understanding patterns of wildlife—spawning seasons for fish, mating and birthing seasons of larger species such as seals and smaller more common water life such as birds—is part of being a wild swimmer. There are chalk valley rivers local to me that I will avoid during spawning season, and I try to avoid nesting swans when swimming in spring.

As well as learning about flora and fauna, it is also good to consider your entry and exit. There is a popular spot on a river near me that swimmers have destroyed by simply entering and exiting the riverbank in the same spot. They raised money to repair it, but not every swimmer is as conscious of their actions.

Tips

— Take your litter home, and also anything else you find while swimming

— Use eco-friendly sunscreens

— Avoid wearing perfumes and lotions before getting into wild water so as not to harm the native wildlife

— Clean your wetsuit, swimsuit, and equipment between swimming spots to protect biosecurity— ensuring you don't spread species that don't belong from one body of water to another

— Walk, cycle, or use public transportation to get to your swim spot—if you do drive, park with consideration for local residents and the natural environment

Where should I leave my stuff?

If possible, limit the number of valuables you take out with you. If on foot, you will need to pack smarter than if you travel on a bike or by car. Where possible, take your belongings with you in a tow float, at least your phone and keys. Leaving equipment on a beach or riverbank can cause all sorts of issues. Theft, concern for abandoned bags, and animal interference are all issues I have heard from other swimmers; I ensure I don't fall victim to them. A dog running off with your chewy shoes—or, worse, marking its territory on your duffle bag—is not ideal when you're off on a tranquil wild swim. Leave as much as possible in a car or packed out of the way.

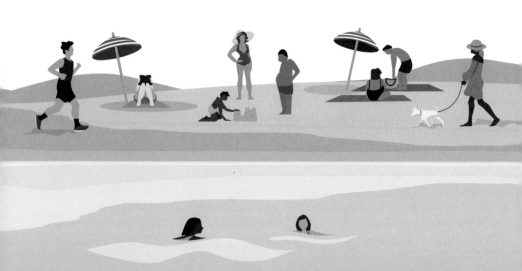

Getting in

Once you have decided where it is safe to enter and exit the water and your equipment is organized for when you get out—you can get in!

Where possible, choose a spot where you can wade into the water gently and consistently. This means that you are moving into the water slowly and not edging in and then stopping, standing, and waiting. Submerge your shoulders, regulate your breathing while still within your depth, and then push off into your swimming stroke. If you're planning on front crawl, try a little breaststroke first to get your body warmed up and used to the water.

If the water you plan to enter is deep, or off a ledge or steps, slide in slowly and hold onto the edge or a float while you regulate your breathing and tread water to warm up.

Once you are in and acclimated to the water, and have seen and experienced the pull, current, tide, and depth, you can start to experiment and jump in, and be more playful.

How long, how far?

Wild swimming is enjoyable because of the freedom of being able to swim for as long or as little as you like. You don't have to fit into a pool schedule! But often I am asked, "How long should I spend in the water?", or "How far should I swim?" What you can achieve in open water each time really does depend on conditions and how you feel on the day. But as long as you are feeling fit, well, and warm, you can swim for as long as you like. In winter, limit your time in colder temperatures and watch out for the cold-water risks (see pages 104–109). Ensure you are well hydrated in warmer conditions. You only need a short swim to get the benefits of cold water. Like any exercise, a regular 30-minute swim is a good goal if conditions allow. A marathon swim in open water is set at 6.2 miles (10 km), and often a good beginner long-distance goal is 1.2 miles (2 km).

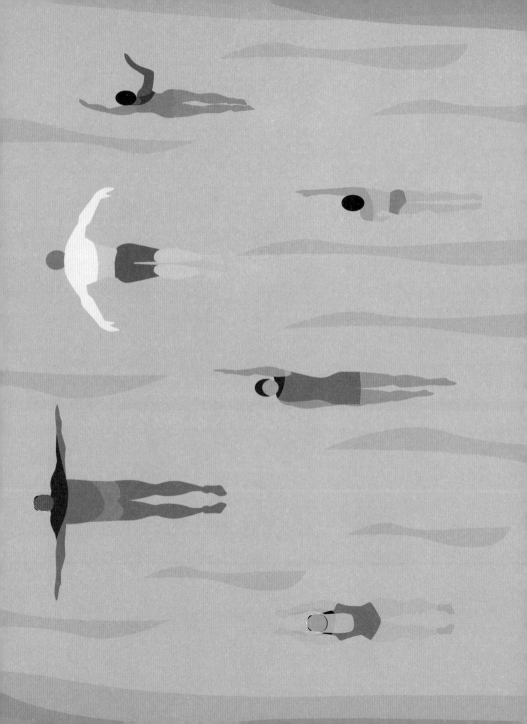

11

SWIMMING STROKES AND SKILLS

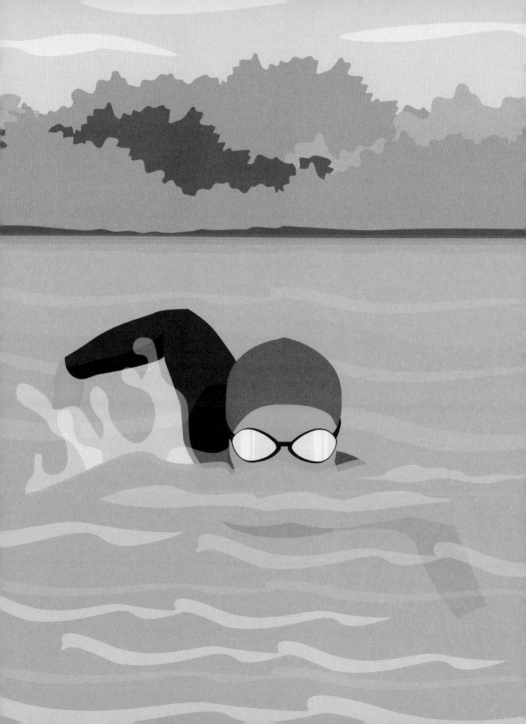

WILD SWIMMING TECHNIQUES

Wild water doesn't care if you swim with your head up using the breaststroke, if you get your head in and crawl, or you lay on your back, eyes to the sky. Swim your own way. It is more important to be safe, comfortable, and aware than to display Olympic-level swimming skills.

One of the joys of outdoor swimming is that it slows us down and immerses us in nature, releasing stress and tension. But sometimes swimming in certain types of water or in trickier conditions demands a stronger stroke, and at times our sense of adventure and curiosity leads us across lakes, down rivers, and between lands. Once you have spent some time in wild water, it is common to want to improve your swimming or set a

goal. It seems a human condition to want to stretch and aspire to something. Lots of issues with swimming are rooted in poor technique. Tire quickly and feel breathless? Your breathing technique needs work. Injury, strains, discomfort? Poor technique. Want to be stronger or faster? Look at your technique!

Each swimming stroke has its advantages in open water. There are also skills you can acquire that will help you adapt to changing conditions. Being able to swim front crawl, as an example, can help you cut through a current better than the breaststroke. How you swim in open water is largely up to you and the conditions you wish to swim in. When starting out, it's best to swim in calm conditions. As in many sports, there are lots of different theories and techniques you can explore. When evaluating the basics of any swimming stroke, a teacher or coach will look at

→ Body position

→ Leg action

→ Arm action

→ Breathing

→ Timing

A combination of these elements is how swimming comes together like magic. They all form part of each stroke.

Breaking down any stroke and working on these elements can be key to improving technique. It helps to work with an open-water coach or swimming teacher—often they can spot things you can't. You could also ask a friend to film you swimming, and see if you can identify where your stroke can be improved. If you don't know where to start, ask yourself how it feels now and how you want it to feel instead. When I first started swimming longer distances in outdoor water, I wanted it to feel effortless rather than exhausting. Let's look at each stroke, common issues with technique, and the style's advantages and disadvantages in wild water.

It is more important to be safe, comfortable, and aware than to display Olympic-level swimming skills.

Front crawl

Crawl is seen as the fastest and most efficient stroke. It is popular in open water, and for good reason. The body position puts a swimmer as flat in the water as possible, which enables a streamlined position that cuts through the water better than other strokes. Front crawl is when you kick your legs continuously, moving your arms in turn out in front of you, pulling the water back to propel you forward.

Advantages

— Fast and efficient

— Enables you to swim in challenging conditions

— Lower risk of injury

— Ideal for swimming longer distances

— Great physical activity

Disadvantages

— Need to learn how to sight in open water (see page 145)

— Miss the view above the water

— Unsociable

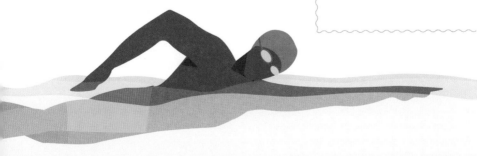

Body position

To achieve the most efficient front crawl, your body should be straight and streamlined in the water. Use a kickboard to practice in a pool or in slow-moving wild water.

1 Place your hands on the kickboard, then straighten your arms out in front of you.

2 Allow your body to rise up behind you, position your face down in the water, and kick your legs. Aim for relaxed shoulders and neck. Your body should be straight and strong.

3 Once comfortable in this position, you can explore breathing (see pages 138–139). Your body position is impacted when you lift your head up out of the water to breathe because your legs drop lower and cause drag, so mastering your breathing technique will help you maintain a good body position.

Leg action

Crawl kicking is simply an up-and-down leg action in a continuous movement. Good technique comes from the hip, with loose knees and flexible ankles.

1 Once your body is in position, practice a gentle kicking action.

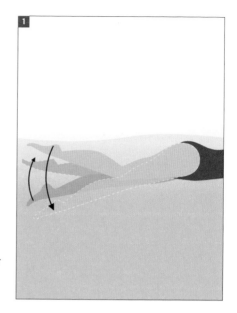

2 Keep your legs and feet just under the surface as you kick using small movements—there is no need for frantic fast kicks. Ensure you are not bending your knees too much—legs should be long and straight out behind you.

Breathing

Mastering your breathing can completely change your front crawl, enabling you to swim farther for longer. Often people hold their breath, or breathe too much or irregularly, when swimming. Taking too much air into your lungs forces you to empty it out

Mastering your breathing can completely change your front crawl, enabling you to swim farther for longer.

too soon. Holding your breath means you need to stop to regulate your breathing again or it can cause panic. Breathing is a foundation to the rhythm of your stroke.

1 Place one hand on top of your kickboard with a straight arm out in front. Put your face in the water and kick your legs (for more detail, see body position and leg action on the preceding page).

2 Place your other arm down by your side and practice rolling the back of your head toward the shoulder of the arm out in front, keeping one ear under the water, and allowing your mouth to reach the surface of the water to take a breath. Blow air out of your nose when your face is in the water, so that when you turn your head, you just need to take a breath in, then turn your head back so that your face is under the water again, and blow out through your nose.

3 Practice with the other arm out in front, using the same technique of rotating the back of your head toward the shoulder of the arm that's out in front, and lifting your face above the surface to take a breath.

In the front crawl, you can breathe every stroke on one side, or every three or five strokes if you're breathing to both sides. Bilateral breathing (when you breathe to both sides) isn't essential, but can be useful. If you are swimming in the sea, for example, and the waves are slapping you in the face every time you try to take a breath, being able to adapt and breathe on the other side can overcome this challenge. Whichever method you choose, avoid holding your breath for too long; this will exhaust you and you won't be able to get into a rhythm because you will need to slow or stop to catch your breath.

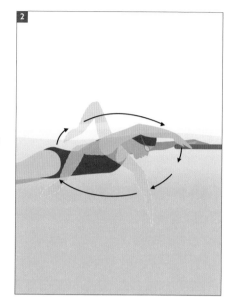

Arm action

Your arms are what pull your body through the water in a crawl—the legs generate only a small amount of propulsion. You essentially want to pull your body past your hand. Often swimmers shorten their pull by cutting their arm into the water too soon, just in front of the head. It is more efficient to reach your arms forward in line with your shoulders and to slice your hands into the water, instead of slapping, enabling a smooth transition into an arm pull.

1   Place one hand on top of your kickboard with a straight arm out in front. With your face down in the water, bring your other arm over your head and out in front, in line with your shoulders and parallel to your straight arm. Keep your fingers together and slightly tilt them as they enter the water in a scooping position, moving down toward your thigh. Before your hand reaches your hip, whip it up out of the water and bring your arm back over your head to repeat the motion.

2   Practice with the other arm, and incorporate the breathing technique. Try to make three arm movements before taking a breath. This will enable bilateral breathing (see page 139). When your arm reaches your hip, turn your head into the rotation to breathe.

Once you have practiced with a kickboard, pull it all together—body position, leg action, breathing, and arm movement—without an aid. Strong, smooth swimming will be more efficient than fast and splashy swimming.

Breaststroke

Heads-up breaststroke is popular among swimmers because you can chat and enjoy the view while you swim. It is also seen as a calm stroke; swimming with your head above water means you can breathe relatively normally. But this doesn't mean you are swimming the stroke in the most efficient way. The breaststroke is a gliding stroke, requiring the same streamlined position as the crawl when not moving your arms and legs. If you can swim heads-down and get into a rhythm of breathing and gliding efficiently, it can be an excellent stroke in wild water. But too much heads-up swimming, chatting, and poor technique can give you neck ache and lower-back problems.

Advantages

— Easy to breathe and keep calm

— Good for warming up the body before entering a different stroke

— Sociable, easy to chat while swimming

— Good visibility

— Great for short swims and dips

— Good to use for a break during the crawl

Disadvantages

— Can impact knees over time

— If not done correctly, it can cause neck and lower back discomfort

— Not efficient in challenging swimming conditions

Body position

To avoid lower-back pain and neck issues, you strive for a horizontal position, especially if you're swimming some distance rather than just dipping and chatting.

1 Lift up into a swim position, with your tummy facing down, legs behind you, and arms out in front. For the more efficient heads-down swimming, your face should be below the surface of the water, except when breathing. At a minimum, try to place your chin on the surface of the water.

Arm action

When learning, practice the arm movement before introducing the legs. Find yourself a pool noodle—a long foam float—to help you.

1 Place the noodle under your tummy so that you can focus on your arms without sinking.

2 Move your arms forward, hands together into an extended straight position out in front of you, then separate both arms outward with fingers together in a scooping position, pushing the water downward and out in a circular motion. Before your arms go behind you, past the hip, bring your hands back together in front of you at the chest, before pushing forward into the extended straight position.

Leg action

With breaststroke the momentum comes from the leg kick. It is called a frog kick, so look at a frog and how it kicks to get an idea of this motion. Often, I see swimmers with one leg that doesn't behave—it takes practice to get the symmetry and get strength in the kick in both legs at the same time. Practice is the best way to resolve this.

1 Practice the leg motion while on your back at first. Using a noodle, place it behind you and lean onto it on your back, with legs extended and together.

2 Move your heels up toward your bottom and turn your feet outward. Push your flexed feet out and around, before bringing your legs back together into a straight-legged glide. Think bend, open legs straight out wide, and then snap legs back together into a glide. Both legs should move together, mirroring each other.

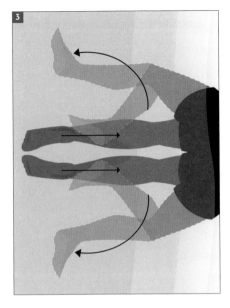

Breathing

In breaststroke you can breathe with each stroke to establish a rhythm. If you don't put your head into the water, for example during winter I find the water too cold for my head, just make sure you keep your head low, chin to the water, neck relaxed.

1   As your arms come into your chest, lift your head out of the water and breathe in.

2   When you push your hands forward to extend your arms, put your face in the water to breathe out. Your neck and shoulders should remain relaxed and long; swimming should be strong and calm, not tight and fast.

3   After practicing on your back, turn over and practice on your tummy. Continue to use the noodle for support if needed.

Once you have the bend, open, and snap movement, you can look at working your legs together with your arms. The arms and legs work in tandem, the arm propulsion followed by the leg kick as arms recover, and then legs and arms move into a streamlined position for the glide. Think arms circle, kick legs open, and then glide into a straight body position.

Backstroke

Butterfly

This isn't a common stroke for open water because you can't see where you are going! There are no markers in the sky like you might find in a pool building to help you visually. This is not a stroke suitable for water busy with other water users, or bending, twisting rivers! That said, swimming on your back is a joy in open water. It allows you to gaze up at the clouds, stars, or treetops. Laying on your back, eyes to the sky, legs kick up and down as in the front crawl. Arms move in a backward motion, one at a time. It is lovely to practice occasionally with awareness of what is around you, and it can be helpful as it allows you to calm your breathing.

This impressive-looking, high-energy stroke can be done in open water with pleasure, but it isn't common. There are records of people swimming butterfly across channels; and in Cambridge, England, the swimmers do butterfly under bridges to scare away trolls! Unless you have learned in a pool and enjoy the stroke, I wouldn't worry too much about it in wild water. If you can swim butterfly, it is fantastic in the sea because you are more buoyant and can roll your body with the movement of the water. Try it if you can!

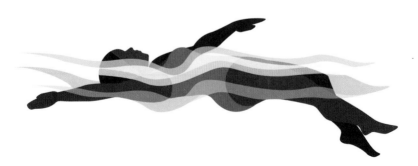

Specific open-water skills

The more you swim in wild water, the more you might seek specific skills to help with personal goals like swimming distance or at speed. There are some particular open-water skills that can help with more ambitious goals in the water—for example, buoy turns in events, where you can change direction around a floating marker. When starting out it is better to keep it simple, but here is one skill that will definitely be useful.

Sighting

When swimming the front crawl in wild water, unlike in a pool, there are no visual markers under the water to help you swim in a straight line or in the direction you wish to swim. In wild water it is useful to sight, which is a technique where you use your surroundings to help you swim on track. In simple terms, sighting is just looking every few strokes at a chosen point in your sightline to ensure you are swimming toward it. Sighting can be part of the breathing movement with the front crawl (see page 139). Everyone has their own way,

but it is easiest to sight just before you take a breath or just after. I find I naturally sight after I take a breath, looking at a chosen marker just before I put my face back in the water.

1 Choose a fixed point or object in the distance in the direction you want to swim. For example, tall trees on the skyline, tops of buildings, beach groins, or flags.

2 Start your front crawl in the direction of your fixed point. After a few strokes, when ready to breathe, lift your eyes a little and glimpse at your chosen point before turning your head to breathe. Then repeat after another few strokes. Adjust your direction to keep on track.

3 Try breathing and looking on both sides, but you might find it easier to sight before breathing on one side in particular. Practice this skill until it becomes second nature and part of your stroke.

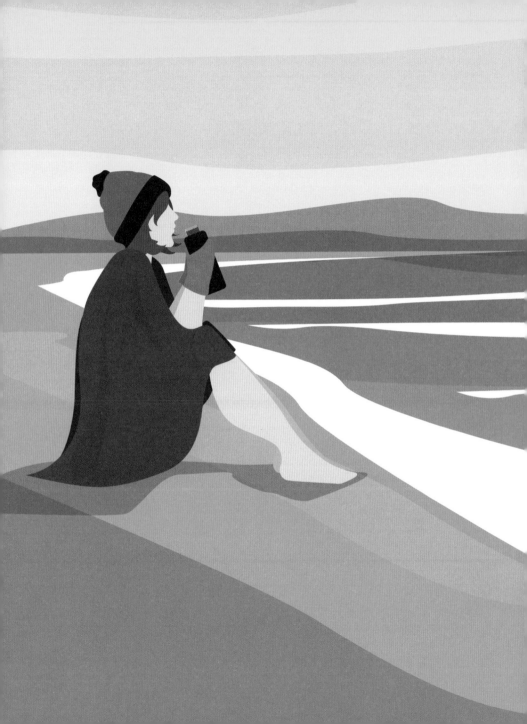

12

AFTER-SWIM CARE

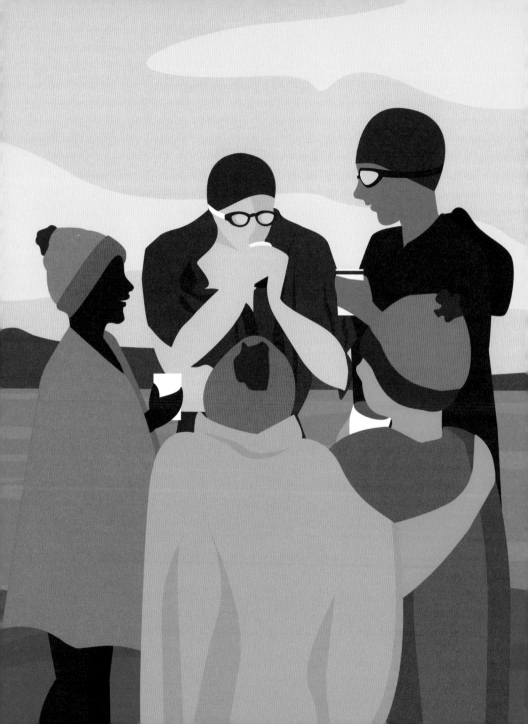

GETTING OUT

Looking after yourself once you get out of the water is every bit as important as the planning and consideration before your swim. While after-swim care may seem as simple as getting dry and dressed, there are some common mistakes that many people make once they leave the water. Having a hot shower or bath after a cold swim, for example, isn't as good as it sounds. Let's explore why and look at more effective after-swim habits.

Drying off and dressing

Like much of the wild swim experience, how you exit and care for yourself after a swim depends on the conditions, weather, and season. After being in outdoor water your body will continue to cool, and being damp can make things worse, even in hot weather. Water evaporating off your skin is a fast way to lose heat, which is why you can feel chilly after a swim, even on a hot day. This is why it's always advisable to dry off and remove wet items in hot conditions as well as cold.

Once dry, get dressed or put on some layers. If you are hanging around the water for a while to enjoy time socially, get warm first. You can always take clothes off again if you want a double dip! Or if you are doing a day of swimming, put on a spare, dry swimsuit before putting clothes on, so that you are ready for your next dip. In cold weather conditions, a thermal base layer, decent sweater, and wind/waterproof coat are must-haves after cold swims. Wool socks are the only

What's in my duffel bag?

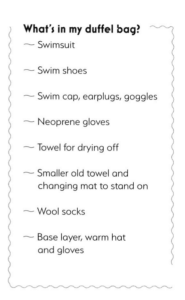

- Swimsuit

- Swim shoes

- Swim cap, earplugs, goggles

- Neoprene gloves

- Towel for drying off

- Smaller old towel and changing mat to stand on

- Wool socks

- Base layer, warm hat and gloves

thing that can warm my toes back to life after cold swims. Changing robes are useful if it is raining or windy because they can keep you warmer while you change under them. But if it is challenging and you find yourself fumbling around for too long, it might be easier to just dry off and get dressed quickly.

Showers and baths

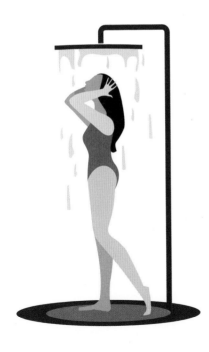

When I first started swimming in the winter, I began in an outdoor pool. It was about 43°F (6°C) in the water, and when I got out, I headed straight to the showers and stood under the pounding hot water. Not only did it burn my skin like it was boiling, but I also soon felt faint and odd. I had to sit down. The lifeguard told me he pulls more people out of the showers in winter than he does out of the pool. Hot showers, tubs, and baths seem like a great idea, but they can open the blood vessels in the skin too quickly, which causes blood to rush out from your core and can lead to a drop in blood pressure, light-headedness, and fainting. The biggest danger then is that you slip and hurt yourself. Another risk is that you can't feel how hot the water really is because your skin is cold and numb, so you could burn yourself. It can also cause itchy discomfort on the skin surface if you try to warm up too quickly. The best way to warm up after swimming is slowly, at the rate you cooled down. Get dry and dressed, have a warm drink, perhaps something to eat, and this will help you warm at a better rate. Once you feel warmer, then you can head to the showers. If you do have a shower or bath, use very tepid water to begin with and bring up the heat of the water slowly as your skin begins to warm.

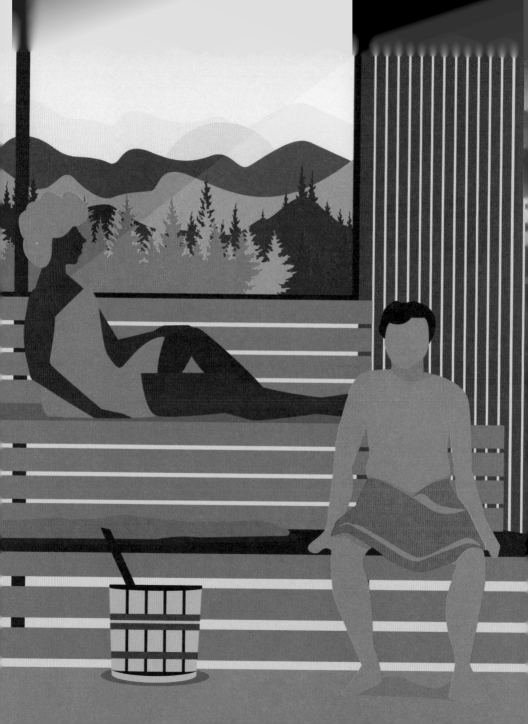

Saunas

Food and drink

Finnish people love saunas, and for good reason. The many benefits are similar to those of wild swimming, so if you sauna before and after a swim, it is super-beneficial. Unlike taking a hot shower, it is safe to sauna before getting in the water and after your cold swim. The warmth in a sauna comes from the air rather than water, as in a shower. Air has less heat energy than water, and so it is safe to have warm air around you to recover. Spending time in the heat and then the cold before returning to the heat is a positive way of stimulating your circulatory and immune systems.

It is common advice to have a hot drink after a cold swim. The idea is that it warms you up from the inside, but scientifically it does very little to your core body temperature. What it does do is replace lost fluids, hydrating the body. It's also a psychological comfort, and holding a warm drink can help warm your fingers. Also, if the warm drink is high energy, like sweet tea or hot chocolate, it will aid recovery as it takes a lot of energy to rewarm your body.

Being hungry after swimming is common, even after pool swimming. Ultimately, it is because you are using energy to exercise, as with any other physical activity, but if you're swimming in cold water you will use even more energy to keep your body warm. Eating after swimming is great—something sweet is ideal if you feel cold, but something warm is even better.

If you sauna before and after a swim, it is super-beneficial.

Top 20 places to wild swim

The world is full of amazing places to swim and this list is by no means exhaustive, but here are some favorites.

Aguelmam Azegza National Park, Morocco
Clear, blue, and cool lakes are located across this beautiful mountain region. It's worth heading into the Atlas Mountains to escape the usual tourist traps in popular coastal areas.

Akigawa River, Akigawa Valley, Japan
Visit in fall to enjoy the spectacular colors of the trees while dipping and paddling in this cool river. If it's too cool, nearby Seoto-no-Yu Spa offers warmer waters.

Bhatta Falls, Mussoorie, India
Deep pool at the bottom of a waterfall. Very popular, but fantastic fun with family or friends.

Bimmah Sinkhole, Qurayyat, Oman
Turquoise mix of sea water and fresh water makes this a stunning swim. Steps into the sinkhole make it easy if not strange to swim in.

Bagni Regina Giovanna, Sorrento, Italy
Swim in the ruins of a Roman villa. Secluded beach and an arch to swim through. Beautiful underwater world to see while cooling off.

Bondi Icebergs Pool, Sydney, Australia
Iconic and stunning, this outdoor pool on Bondi Beach offers excellent swimming lanes with the wild coastline backdrop.

Brighton Beach, New York, USA
Swim where movies have been made and walk the boardwalk. In winter, join the Coney Island Polar Bear swimmers.

Camps Bay, Cape Town, South Africa
Fine white sand, natural rock pool, and views of the Twelve Apostles mountains. Swimming in this clear water is like swimming in an aquarium, with amazing wildlife and visibility.

Cenotes, Tulum, Mexico
Incredible swimming holes and caves in Mexico that will mesmerize you. Truly wild and adventurous swimmers, get some local knowledge or, even better, a local guide.

Cleopatra's Pool, Pamukkale, Turkey
Although a managed facility, this is famous for the wild and wonderful offer of dips and swims. Geothermal water and old Roman ruins to swim under and around.

Crystal Bay, Bali, Indonesia
There are many great places to swim in Indonesia, but this is a favorite for encounters with turtles and for snorkeling. Crystal-clear water gave it its name.

Hampstead Ponds, London, England
Swim wild in Central London—yes really! Deep, dark ponds popular with locals are jammed in a heatwave and peaceful in the rain. Swim with ducks and under weeping willows.

Isle of Arran, Scotland
Sea, river pools, and mountain lochs: the Isle of Arran has it all for adventurous swimmers. Swim with seals and then warm up with whisky afterward.

Lake of Sainte-Croix, France
Turquoise water, rocks to leap and dive from, boats to rent, and beaches to sunbathe on. Worth a trip into the mountains.

Lake Zurich, Switzerland
At 25 miles (40km) long, this blue, cool-water lake has wonderful access and facilities all around it. At the city end, bathe from wooden platforms that offer food, drink, and sundecks.

Park forest Zlatni Rt, Rovinj, Croatia
Tranquil park with cedar trees, white pebble beaches, and crystal-clear water. Walk, cycle, or picnic waterside among the wildlife.

Pescadores Beach, Lima, Peru
Scenic views in an artisanal fishing port and tranquil waters to swim in, adjacent to the capital of Peru.

Rauhaniemen kansankylpylä, Tampere, Finland
In summer, enjoy swimming in a gorgeous lake with easy access. In winter, swim in an ice hole and warm up in the folk sauna.

Sitka National Historical Park, Alaska, USA
Swim with salmon and sea lions along the coast of this beautiful national park. Take a boat out to one of the many islands for a remote swim.

Terra Nostra Park in Furnas, São Miguel Island, Azores
Natural thermal water pools in a stunning botanical garden. Steeped in history and beauty, the location offers warm, wild water from the ground.

Seek local advice and information before swimming at any of these locations!

Index

A

access issues 69
after-swim care 147–53
afterdrop 108
air temperature 95, 99
algae 112–13
apps, wild swimming 71
arms: breaststroke 142
    front crawl 140
    treading water 34–5
arthritis 62

B

backstroke 144
bare feet 60
baths 151
beaches 82
belongings, where to leave 130
benefits of wild swimming 14–20
bicycle kick 33
bikinis 41–2
blue-green algae 113
board shorts 43
boats, risks 97
bodies of water 79–89
body temperature 104,
    106–8, 110
body types 17
breaststroke 141–3
    treading water 33, 35
breathing: breaststroke 143
    cold water shock 104
    front crawl 138–9
    sighting 145
briefs 43
bruises 108–9
buoyancy shorts 43
Burgess, Thomas 54
bust support, swimsuits 41
butterfly stroke 144

C

cameras, waterproof 65
cancer, skin 110
caps 52–3
Carr, Karen Eva 13
changing mats 65

changing robes 63, 150
chop, sea swimming 82, 120
cold water shock 104, 119
cold-water swimming 20,
    104–9, 120
communities 72
costs 17
cotton/nylon fabric swim
    caps 53
cramps 108
crawl, front 137–40
crawl kick, treading water 33
crocs 60
currents 96, 99
cuts 108–9
cyanobacteria 113

D

dark, swimming in 121
Daws, Vanessa 20
depth of water 96, 99
dressing 150
drinks 153
drowning chain 94
dry suits 45
drying off 63, 150

E

earplugs 54, 109
ear problems 13, 54, 109
Ederle, Gertrude 54
egg beater technique 32
electrical storms 119
English Channel 45, 54
entry and exit points 71, 82, 85–6,
    87, 89, 95, 99, 131
environmental issues 16, 129
equinoxes 122
equipment 49–65

F

fabrics, swimsuits 42
fall swimming 120
fear of water 25
feet 60–61, 96, 99
first-aid kits 65
fitness 27
fjords 87
flip-flops 60
floating 29–31

floats 59, 130
flow, risks 86, 96, 99
fog 118
food and drink 153
footwear 60–61
front crawl 137–40

G

gadgets 65
gasp reaction 104
getting into water 131
getting out of water 149
gloves 60, 62
goggles 54–7
groups 72
guidebooks 71

H

hands, gloves 60, 62
Harper, Dr. Mark 20
hats 53, 109
hazards 86, 96, 99, 109
health 14, 97, 99
heatstroke 110, 119
hijabs 44
hot-water swimming 110–13
hyperthermia 95, 110
hypothermia 95, 106–7

I, J

ice swimming 121
indoor pools 28, 89, 151
infections 13, 54, 57,
    60, 109
inner child 15
instincts, trusting 94
ions, negative 14
isolation 19
itch, swimmer's 113
jammers 43
jellyfish 80, 96
Jones, Lucy 14

K, L

knit hats 53
lakes 69, 75, 79, 87
latex swimming caps 52
laws 75
learning to swim 25, 26
leggings 44

legs: breaststroke 142
  front crawl 138
  treading water 32–3
lifeguards 75, 82, 89, 94, 151
lightning 119
lights, waterproof 65
litter 16, 86, 96, 97, 117, 129
lochs 87
loneliness 19

M
maps 70–71
mats, changing 65
mental health 14
microfiber towels 63
mitigating risks 98–9
modest swimwear 44
moon, phases of 122
muscles: cramping 108
  swim failure 105

N, O
negative ions 14
neoprene: gloves 62
  socks 61
  swim caps 52
  wetsuits 45, 110
night swimming 65, 121–2
open-water venues 75
outdoor pools 8, 89

P
panic 25, 104, 108, 112
parasites, swimmer's itch 113
parks 75
planning 128–30
plants 96, 99, 112–13
pollution 16, 86, 95, 97, 99
ponds 79, 87
pools 79, 89
preparations 125–31
prescription goggles 57
public spaces 75

R
rainfall 86, 87, 118
research 70–71
reservoirs 87
resilience 20
Reynaud's 62

risks 93–9
river pools 89
rivers 69, 79, 85–6, 95, 96
robes 63, 150
rubber swim caps 53
rules 16, 69, 75

S
safety 19, 72, 91–9
saunas 153
scissor kick 33
sculling 34–5
sea swimming 69, 79, 80–82, 122
  risks 95, 96, 99
seals 80, 96
seasons 115–22
sensory experiences 20
shock, cold water 104, 119
shoes 60
shorts 43
shower shoes 60
showers 151
sighting 145
silicone: earplugs 54
  swimming caps 52
skills, specific 145
skin: cancer 110
  cuts and bruises 108–9
"skins" swimmers 45, 46
sliders 60
snow 121
social media 71, 72
socks 60–61, 150
solstices 122
Sotelo, Ana Elisa 19
speed of rivers 86
spring swimming 117, 118
star floats 30–31
storms 119
strength 20
stress 20
strokes 133–44
summer swimming 103, 119
sun exposure 110, 119
sunrise and sunset 122
surfer's ear 109
swell, sea swimming 81, 120
swim caps 52–3
swim failure 105
swim fitness 27

swim gear 49–65
swimmer's ear 13, 109
swimmer's itch 113
swimming, learning 25, 26
swimming pools 28, 89
swimming shoes 61
swimming strokes 133–44
swimsuits 17, 41–2
swimwear 39–47

T, U
tarns 87
temperatures 95, 99, 103–13
thunder 119
tidal pools 89
tidal rivers 85
tides 80–81, 95, 96, 99, 122
tow floats 59, 130
towels 63
treading water 32–5
triathlons 45–6
  Las Truchas 19
trunks 43
underwater hazards 86, 109
UV protection 42, 110

W
watches, waterproof 65
water quality 95, 99
water shoes 61
water temperature 95, 99
water users, safety 97, 99
waterfalls 40, 86, 89
waves, sea swimming 81, 120
weather 86, 87, 95, 99
weeds 112
weirs 86, 89
wetsuits 39, 40, 45–7, 110
where to swim 69–75, 154–5
whistles 65
wildlife 129
  risks 95, 96, 99
  in rivers 86
  sea swimming 80
wind, fall swimming 120
winter swimming 103, 117, 121

Further reading

I hope that most questions you might have had about wild swimming have been covered in the book, but you might be interested in reading more or developing your knowledge. Here are some suggested titles that can enhance your wild swimming further.

Books

Waterlog, Roger Deakin (Vintage, 1999)

Haunts of the Black Masseur—The Swimmer as a Hero, Charles Sprawson, (Vintage, 1992)

The Outdoor Swimmers' Handbook, Kate Rew (Ebury Publishing, 2022)

Shifting Currents—A World History of Swimming, Karen Eva Carr (Reaktion Books, 2022)

Swim Wild and Free—A Practical Guide to Swimming Outdoors 365 Days a Year, Simon Griffiths (Bloomsbury, 2022)

Chill: The Cold Water Swim Cure, Dr. Mark Harper (Chronicle Books, 2022)

How to Read Water: Clues & Patterns from Puddles to the Sea, Tristan Gooley (Hodder & Stoughton, 2016)

Websites

→ www.outdoorswimmer.com
→ www.thedipadvisor.co.uk
→ www.outdoorswimmingsociety.com
→ www.fina.org
→ www.openwaterswimming.com

Acknowledgments

From the author

There are several swimmers and people who have influenced, educated, supported, and inspired me over the years. Much of my experience and knowledge I owe to the people I have swam with over my life—so thank you to you all. Special thanks to Jeni Orme, who has swum alongside me in all seasons and all conditions right from the beginning when the idea of river swimming was still seen as insane. Thanks to Roger Taylor and Deb Phillips for being swim idea testers, great friends, and willing swim explorers. Thank you to swim teachers, coaches, and guides who have taken me for a swim, taught me to swim better, and helped me learn how to help others. Of course, none of my swimming would have been possible without my Mum and Dad, who not only enabled swimming lessons at a young age, but who have also been wild swimming with me my whole life. Love and thanks to Bruno and Hugo, who are always willing to walk through mud, wind, and rain, up and down hills, and picnic in the elements, hold my towel, and leap in and swim with me no matter what.

From the publisher

The publisher would like to thank John Friend for proofreading and Hilary Bird for indexing. DK would also like to thank the following for permission to include extracts on the pages cited below:

→ p16; Simon Griffiths for insight from *Outdoor Swimmer* magazine

→ p19; Ana Sotelo and IWPA, "Las Truchas: A School of Women"

→ p20; from *Chill*, ©2022 Mark Harper. Used with Permission from Chronicle Books, LLC. Visit www.ChronicleBooks.com.

→ p20; From the film "At Home in the Water," 2022, by artist Vanessa Daws

About the author

Ella Foote is Director and Founder of Dip Advisor—an outdoor swim guiding company offering swim experiences in wild and open-water locations. A renowned swimming journalist, Ella writes for UK media, and has appeared on several podcasts and television programs. She's also Editor of *Outdoor Swimmer* magazine, is an RLSS Open Water Lifeguard, STA Open Water Coach, and STA Swim Teacher. An intrepid swim explorer, she is constantly seeking out new rivers, lakes, ponds, seas, and pools to plunge into. She enjoys swimming in all seasons and has completed swims such as an English Channel relay crossing, 24-hour swim challenge, the Thames Marathon 14k, and the Dart 10k, as well as smaller, more joyful dips and dunks across the world.

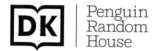

Penguin Random House

DK LONDON
Project Editor Lucy Philpott
US Editor Lori Cates Hand
Senior Designer Tania Gomes
Senior Acquisitions Editors Zara Anvari, Becky Alexander
Senior Production Editor Tony Phipps
Production Controller Rebecca Parton
Jacket Coordinator Abi Gain
Editorial Manager Ruth O'Rourke
Art Director Maxine Pedliham
Publishing Director Katie Cowan

Project Editor Emma Hill
Designer Sarah Pyke
Illustrator Luisa Tosetto

First American Edition, 2023
Published in the United States by DK Publishing
1745 Broadway, 20th Floor, New York, NY 10019

Text copyright © Ella Foote 2023
Copyright © 2023 Dorling Kindersley Limited
A Division of Penguin Random House LLC
23 24 25 26 27   10 9 8 7 6 5 4 3 2 1
001–335370–Nov/2023

A catalog record for this book
is available from the Library of Congress.
ISBN: 978-0-7440-8448-1

Printed and bound in China

For the curious
www.dk.com